FROM DEPRESSION TO WHOLENESS

THE ANATOMY OF HEALING

Debbie Thurman

Foreword by Bettie B. Youngs, Ph.D.

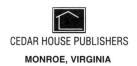

CEDAR HOUSE PUBLISHERS

MONROE, VIRGINIA

From Depression to Wholeness: The Anatomy of Healing
Copyright © 2000 by Deborah M. Thurman

Requests for information should be addressed to:

Cedar House Publishers
P. O. Box 399
Monroe, Virginia 24574-0399
Cedarhousepub@aol.com

ISBN: 0-9676289-0-3
Library of Congress Card Catalog Number: 99-096106

All Scripture quotations, unless otherwise indicated, are taken from the Holy Bible, New International Version®. NIV®. Copyright 1973, 1978, 1984 by International Bible Society. Used by permission of Zondervon Publishing House. All rights reserved.

Scripture also taken from the NEW AMERICAN STANDARD BIBLE, © 1960, 1962, 1963, 1968, 1971, 1972, 1973, 1975, 1977, by The Lockman Foundation. Used by permission. Other Scripture from the King James Version.

All rights reserved. No part of this publication may be reproduced, stored in a retrieval system or transmitted in any form or by any means — electronic, mechanical, photocopy, recording or any other — except for brief quotations in reviews, without the prior, written permission of the publisher.

Printed in the United States of America
Cover and interior design by The Design Group and Russ Thurman
Cover photograph by Russ Thurman

For Russ
and for Jenni and Natalie,
who are the apples of my eyes.

*To Sonja —
May God bless you!
Debbie Shuman
3/2/02*

Most of the grand truths of God have to be burned into us with the hot iron of affliction, otherwise we shall never truly receive them.

C.H. Spurgeon

Sure I am that this day we are masters of our fate, that the task which has been set before us is not above our strength; that its pangs and toils are not beyond my endurance. As long as we have faith in our own cause and an unconquerable will to win, victory will not be denied us.

Winston Churchill

And I will restore to you the years that the locust hath eaten ... And ye shall eat in plenty, and be satisfied, and praise the name of the LORD your God that hath dealt wondrously with you.

Joel 2:25-26 (KJV)

Acknowledgments

I owe my deepest gratitude to some special people for their assistance in getting this book into print. First, I am grateful to my husband, Russ and to my daughters, Jenni and Natalie, for allowing me the time to research and write it and for encouraging me when the going got tough.

I must thank the following people who took the time to read developing drafts: Rev. Rick and Vonnie Savage, my mother Lourine Massie, Carol Scamara, Pam Martin, Claudia Nardone, Janet Alvarado, Colleen Hughes, Sherwood E. Wirt, Dr. Bernie Siegel, Carol LeBeau, Merry Falduti, Drs. Les and Leslie Parrott and my husband, who is a wonderful editor and publisher. Russ, we *are* the A-team.

A special heartfelt thank-you goes to Bettie Youngs and to Jerry Freed, who helped me turn the corner and wouldn't let me quit. Gratitude and "hugs" to my agent, Barbara Neighbors Deal, for her cheery, upbeat attitude and for making me smarter. I am also deeply grateful to those who checked my writing at various times for technical accuracy: Dr. R. Bruce Hubbard, Diane M. Eller-Boyko, R.N., LCSW and John L. Sexton, Ph.D., ABPP, Commander, MSC, U.S. Navy.

I am especially grateful to Rev. and Mrs. Jerry Falwell, who took time from an enormously busy schedule to read the manuscript and give their support and encouragement to "win and win big."

My hat is off to Scott Kirkwood of The Design Group in Lynchburg, Virginia for his creativity and his patience with me, even when confronted with yet another dumb question.

Thanks to the Sweet Briar College Library for their assistance with Interlibrary Loan and archived materials.

Last, I thank my Lord and Savior, Jesus Christ, who gives me hope, reproof, guidance, wisdom, grace and love throughout each and every day.

Contents

Foreword	xi
Introduction	xiii
1. "Why Art Thou Cast Down, O My Soul?"	1
2. My Parents' Child	21
3. The Anatomy Of Depression	35
4. A Heart's Quest	63
5. I'm Okay, You're Okay ... Aren't We?	77
6. "Amor Vincit Omnia"	97
7. Words Of Love And Healing	119
8. I've Got To Be Me, But Who Am I?	133
9. No Greater Love	145
10. Instruments of Healing	155
11. Lessons From The Scribes	171
Epilogue	193
Appendix: Ten Tips For Conquering Depression	197
Notes	201
Where to Get Information and Help	207

Foreword

It is a sad fact in this age of medical breakthroughs that an estimated 17-20 million Americans suffer from clinical depression, either episodic or chronic. Doctors say that two-thirds of these receive no treatment and that countless more are dealing with emotional precursors that will lead to full-blown clinical depressive disorders if left untreated. In record numbers people feel that a great chasm separates them from all that is meaningful. This pain is real, as is their despair over believing there is no way of ever crossing the turbulent, ominous waters to reach a state of wellness, wholeness and true happiness.

How can we best heal those experiencing depression's destructiveness and how might we prevent others from falling into the quagmire in the first place? Does the answer lie in the scientific world? Or is the prescription more readily found in the field of counseling, or in the church? Who is to say?

Depression is a very complex agenda, a mysterious imbalance between the psyche and soma, mind and body. We know so much, and yet so little. There's a chance we'll never find the key to unlock this secret, sacred door to health and wholeness, though this book is a step in the right direction. This remarkable book is, in part, a highly graphic account of Debbie Thurman's decade-long experience with undiagnosed Major Depressive Disorder (MDD) and five subsequent years of treatment following that diagnosis. Indeed, Debbie looked behind every door in her search for a life-line that might help her return to a life worth living. As it is for most, her bout with depression was a long and excruciating journey, one that snatched her from the light of day, plummeted her into the depths of darkness, and for many years pummeled her before finally releasing her back to the light.

But this book is more than the telling of a personal trial, tribulation and then triumph over circumstance. It is a prescription of sorts — a prescription for what ails so many of us at the soul level. Though you may or may not draw the same conclusions Debbie Thurman does, you will discover many truths in the search for wholeness. If you seek practical, tried-by-fire remedies, they are here. For those who like statistics and science, the author does not disappoint, culling the best from the ongoing research in depressive illnesses. As for the relationship between science and theology — one that often gets short shrift by those trying to bring us answers — she has successfully bridged this gap, too. Moreover, she has given us the tools with which to examine it for ourselves.

Debbie Thurman is Everyman, Everywoman, as robust and fragile as any of us. But like the tender shoot pushing through the cold, hard soil that she describes in this book's epilogue, she affirms the resiliency of humanity and reminds us that we are all but "plantings of the Lord," ever growing, hence profoundly worthy of whole lives. As the author so aptly builds a case, the journey is to deepen into our limitations — so that we might delight in the discovery that this is where our wholeness, our essence comes from. In this there is real freedom.

Bettie B. Youngs, Ph.D.
Author, *Taste-Berry Tales* and
A String of Pearls: Inspirational Stories on the Resiliency of the Human Spirit

Introduction

I've always been supremely interested in people and what makes them who they are. From my youth, I set out to become a journalist so that I could chronicle the lives of people around me and the events that shape them. I remember being influenced by reading Anne Frank's diary, wherein she confessed "I want to go on living even after my death! And therefore I am grateful to God for giving me this gift, this possibility of developing myself and of writing, of expressing all that is in me."[1] It never occurred to me that one day I'd be observing my own life under a clinical microscope — that I'd be chronicling the illness of my own mind.

We humans do our utmost to avoid or control pain, yet pain is an unavoidable part of life. Perhaps we should embrace it instead, and try to learn what it is teaching us. Even in many of our churches, suffering is no longer theologically correct. Some of us tend to brush aside the suffering soul or feed it healthy doses of joy and positive thinking without first acknowledging the sacredness in sorrow. "Will not the deepening darkness brighten the glimmering star?" assures my late grandfather's favorite, old gospel hymn. There is no great shame in experiencing depression. Many have been there. It's not a place that we need to stay, however.

I know the extent of the suffering that depressed people endure. It is, in a word, hell. I know, too, the pain of watching family members suffer from depressive disorders and other forms of mental illness. My father and one of my brothers spent years in mental hospitals undergoing treatment for bipolar disorder as well as schizophrenia, all compounded by substance abuse. My father recovered; my brother has yet to do so. One allowed himself to be utterly broken and rebuilt anew. The other remained defiant and wouldn't — or couldn't — acknowledge his brokenness.

Where does depression originate? To what extent can we alter this condition and what forces control it? Coming to terms with these questions can change the way we cope with and ultimately find healing from the "dark night of the soul." Depression is a biological, psychological and spiritual disorder that, for each individual, may take some time to fully deal with depending upon its severity and causes. The external *modus vivendi* — possible medication, diet, exercise (both physical and mental) — are important, but are not ends in themselves. Relief can come rather quickly. Honest assessment and true healing will take longer, but they're worth the journey, as I found out first-hand. No one will recover fully from major depression without some kind of communal support system. Religious communities and families are ideally suited to provide this support. No matter where you start, ultimately you will have to look up to higher ground. The answer is neither exclusively within you or around you. It is, for the most part, *above* you.

While I have overcome much, I am still after all, a vulnerable human being. I'm not perfectly healed. I simply see myself as the recipient of God's perfect grace, in the right amounts and at the right times. That grace now becomes what Pastor/Counselor David Seamands calls "recycling grace" or healing grace that is passed along to others. I am truly grateful for the healing touch of the Great Physician, as well as that of the physicians and counselors He appointed for me. I speak from my experience as a Christian, though I live in a world where Judeo-Christian mores coexist with other value systems.

In the past year or two, public and media attention have been unusually focused on the relationship between our spiritual and emotional health. We are looking for answers. Too many bruised and battered people with loose moorings are still drifting away in life's roiling and storm-driven seas. I am but one member of a search and rescue team. If you are treading water, it is my prayer that you will see this book as one of the boats you can use to get to solid ground where answers await you.

Debbie Thurman
Madison Heights, Virginia
November 5, 1999

One

We ought to think that we are one of the leaves of a tree, and the tree is all humanity. We cannot live without the others, without the tree.

Pablo Casals

~~~~~~~~~~~

"Why Art Thou Cast Down, O My Soul?"[1]

I came to know the black beast called the "dark night of the soul" in my mid-twenties when I took a wrong turn that set off a chain of traumatic events in my life. I don't recall being what we term clinically depressed before then, although I believe the beast appeared to me in my childhood.

I have been either cursed or blessed, depending on one's point of view, with great depth of emotion. When I am happy, my joy can soar to the heavens. Likewise, I have known pain that has left me at the very gates of hell. Thankfully, those gates have remained closed. I suspect that has something to do with my learning that it's best to let pain carry you to the threshold of heaven where there is One waiting to absorb it. But as a child, before I learned that truth, I sometimes felt terribly lonely. When I felt unloved, I played a little game wherein I'd fantasize about my own death, complete with the funeral scene where all my family would come and weep over me and say what a wonderful child I'd been. *Suppose I really were to die,* I'd imagine. Then, I believed, they'd all be sorry they ignored me, a slight I felt more deeply than was merited, I'm sure. At times I wanted to trade my pain — the pain of feeling disconnected — for theirs in losing me. Believing in heaven at an early age, I only hoped I'd be in the most wonderful of places after I was gone.

As I reached adulthood, the unexplained sadness and sense of emptiness began to deepen. In college, I was drawn to dark literature or sad tales of unrequited love. After all, those were the stories of my life. As a young Marine journalist/public affairs officer, I pursued an in-depth story on child abuse. I became so absorbed in it, I won an award. I felt an odd kinship with the abusive mother at the center of my story, especially as she spoke of her relationship with her father. I realized that there but for the grace of God went I.

I was newly married, but not particularly happy at this time. I'd married another lieutenant whom I barely knew and with whom I had very little in common. It was one of those whirlwind Officer Candidate School romances that I'd been forewarned about by my advisors. I had thought I was immune. The Marine Corps was experimenting with co-ed training for officers in the late '70s, and everywhere we women went, the cameras were sure to follow. We lived a fairy tale, perpetuated by media hype. (Make no mistake, the physical training *was* real). Since I'd lived at home during my college years, I was like a bird out of a cage, in a co-ed dormitory environment for the first time. I successfully, or so I thought, lived the dual life of squared-away lieutenant by day and occasional party girl by night. I had too few "wild oats" to sow in college, so I bloomed late. In truth, I was still smarting from the jilting I'd received from my high school sweetheart. Consequently, I trapped myself in a marriage I didn't even want. My budding career became the focal point of my life, and my survival tactic. The God of my youth somehow got left out of the picture.

One day, I found myself sitting at my desk in the public affairs office at Camp Lejeune, North Carolina, arranging and rearranging press releases. I couldn't muster the concentration required to edit a single line. My press chief, a kindly master sergeant the troops all adored, noticed my vacant stare and knew something was wrong. I was in a foxhole, in my private war and I couldn't seem to get myself out. He came up and asked to speak with me alone. "Ma'am," he said, "I've seen that kind of look you have in your eyes before." He didn't say where, but I assumed he meant in Vietnam. "Is there anything I can do?" he inquired, with fatherly concern. His gentleness brought me to the verge of tears. "I don't know," was all I could choke out. He said, "If I weren't an enlisted man, I'd give you a hug. I think you need to go home and let your husband do that." He didn't know that I cringed every time my husband embraced me.

My husband and I had been too emotionally immature to marry, but that never seems to stop passion. Our marriage appeared doomed to fail and I wanted out. I couldn't bear to see my life's aspirations snuffed out. I was too closed-minded to seriously consider reconciliation, though I made several half-hearted attempts. It would have been simpler and far less costly if I'd just packed my bags and left. But instead a knight in shining armor rode into the picture. He was a reluctant knight, to be sure, at first gallantly trying to help me save my marriage. Despite our noble attempts at platonic friendship, we fell in genuine love. He was a warrant officer and technically, as a lieutenant, I outranked him. What a joke! He taught me what it meant to be a Marine, including the sacred trust that goes with it, which made the pain of our relationship all the more poignant. He was a poster-perfect, 8th-and-I-Street kind of Marine, ramrod straight with knife-like creases in his uniform and rows of campaign ribbons across his chest, including a Purple Heart from Vietnam. He was a gentleman, this ruggedly handsome "gunner," and a knockout in dress blues. Most importantly, he was an old-fashioned man of substance. Today I am blessed to have shared my life with this wonderful man for 18 years. But the road to our past is littered with debris like so much shrapnel from the land mines the world and our own folly placed in our path.

It was painful to remember that I had actually met Russ Thurman before I had met my then husband. My uncle, a career officer, had arranged for me to tour the public affairs office at Camp Lejeune before I embarked on my officer training. I admit even then I was a bit taken by this lanky gent, but he barely took note of me. He was eight years my senior and to him, I just looked like another bored college kid. I couldn't help looking for him at the Commandant's formal reception I attended. He would have stood out from the young lieutenants whose chests were adorned only by silver shooting badges. But he never showed up. I couldn't help wondering later how the course of my life might have changed had he been there.

When I eventually came to be stationed at Camp Lejeune in the same office with Gunner Thurman, I had only vague recollections of my brief attraction to him the previous year. Nevertheless, I soon found myself wondering what his social life was like. Was he married to the Corps? I soon found out that Russ was greatly admired and respected by seniors and subordinates alike. Folks in the office seemed to band together with great concern over his needs. This led our rather pushy officer-in-charge to coerce me (I was still pretty naïve about this Corps business) into accompanying Russ as a "mercy" date to my first Marine Corps Birthday Ball, traditionally a big event to all Marines. I was not planning to attend because my husband was on a short-term deployment, and Russ was going alone. My husband saw no harm in it, nor did I at the time. We had an innocently great time. But a tiny seed of romance was planted that night.

Later, as Thanksgiving approached, this same protectiveness emerged when a young, married, enlisted woman in the office who had worked in Russ' section asked me one day if my husband and I would consider having him over for the traditional dinner as she and her husband were going to visit relatives for the holiday. She feared he would end up eating alone in the mess hall otherwise. I agreed. In fact, I ended up preparing turkey dinners in two shifts that day to feed not only Russ, but some extra straggler Marines from my husband's unit whom I couldn't fit into my tiny house all at the same time. Thus, a cordial relationship among my husband, Russ and me was born.

In the first meaningful conversation outside any official setting that Russ and I had, I learned that he was married, but had been separated from his wife for seven years. It had been a rocky road for him. My heart went out to Russ because he was keeping his alliance in name only for his children's sake. He spent every Christmas and summer leave with them. Now I understood more of why he evoked compassion from his peers. At this point, we moved from being merely acquaintances to being friends. It just naturally blossomed from there. We seemed to need each other too much. It was painfully sweet and all too romantic for me to walk away. I also was aware that Russ embodied all the positive qualities of my dad. When I met Russ, I felt as if I'd come home.

When my infantry officer husband eventually became aware of what was happening, he was quite naturally enraged. He took his revenge with military precision by mobilizing the Marine Corps mechanism and conducting a heavy, frontal assault on us. We had violated the Corps code of brotherhood, and that couldn't be tolerated. Oh how we knew that all too well! Russ and I lost the ensuing battle, with severe consequences for our careers. An outspoken commanding general with strong moral convictions saw to that. We did win the war — or so it seemed. We had each other, but the real war was just beginning.

I had to walk through the gauntlet of sordid gossip and endure my battalion commander's cold-hearted assessment of Russ' intent, in his opinion, to abandon me to save his career. He couldn't have been more wrong, and I knew it.

I must interject here that I have no intention of romanticizing adultery or of glossing over the fact that we *sinned*. Period. The unpopular word "sin" has been stricken from post-modern usage. Closing our eyes doesn't make the concept of sin go away any more than a toddler can magically make himself disappear in a game of hide and seek. In addition to breaking God's law, the most egregious crime of all, Russ and I stood guilty of violating military law — the Uniform Code of Military Justice (UCMJ). This code is little understood by the civilian world, but I swore an oath to uphold it. There is a great debate today over just what form of punishment is appropriate to service members who discredit good order and discipline by crossing the established moral boundaries of the UCMJ in committing adultery. I'm not sure myself how best to handle these cases, but they can't be ignored. We were rebuked severely because of who we were. As official spokespeople, our military careers put us in the public eye. In order for our command to save face, we had to be pilloried in the square as an example to others who might contemplate such transgressions.

I would never demean all that I hold sacred by hurling bitter invectives at the U.S. Marine Corps, and I have forgiven those who threw stones at us, even though some of them were boulders. Though I was forced to give up my regular commission, I later came back to the Corps and served a tour of duty as a reservist, afterward being honorarily retired as a captain. Russ also went on to retire with dignity as a captain. We'll always be honored to have served our country, despite our blemished records. Without a doubt, I grew up in the Corps. Those were, in the Dickensonian sense, the best of times and the worst of times.

As providence would have it, there was one senior staff officer at Camp Lejeune who had been more concerned with saving my soul than with sparing the image of the Marine Corps. John Grinalds, a soft-spoken lieutenant colonel at the time who was unashamed of his faith, took me aside one day and spoke to me about forgiveness and things eternal. He even prayed with me. I related to him my Christian upbringing. I was aware of how far I'd fallen from grace and I had tears in my eyes when I left his office.

I found out years later when Oliver North came into the spotlight during the Iran-Contra hearings that Grinalds, today a retired major general, was the agent through whom North was healed of a serious back injury during a dramatic prayer session in 1978 following a live-fire exercise at Camp Lejeune. Ollie's response, as General Grinalds today recalls it, was, "My God, Colonel, you've got power!" "No, Ollie, Jesus Christ has power," replied Grinalds. He urged North to think about why Christ had healed him. In the ensuing months, North became a committed Christian. While my turnaround may not have been so dramatic, that prayer took its effect on my life. I never forgot the man or the prayer.

My years in the Marine Corps had a timeless impact on my life. Until recently, I was having occasional dreams at night about being an officer. In every scenario, I was asked to perform a task that I no longer felt capable of doing. But I persevered and came through with accolades each time. In truth, I first recognized my parenting instincts in the Corps. I mothered my troops and felt great compassion for them, but I held them accountable and forced them to grow. They did the same for me. A great Marine general once said that the ideal relationship between a leader and those he or she leads is that of a parent and child. When I actually became a parent, I understood that even more clearly.

After the smoke cleared and Russ was transferred to the West Coast, we tried to settle into some kind of normal life. After my divorce was granted, we were married in a small, simple ceremony by a Navy chaplain. I took a corporate job in San Diego and we bought a house. Try as I may, I couldn't leave the past behind me. I pretended I didn't feel guilty, but I woke in the middle of the night from recurring nightmares of our official trauma. It was Russ the system had really gone after, but I'd sacrificed my career hoping his would be spared. Our reputations as Marines were all but shattered. Many chinks in my first husband's armor (as well as for those who judged us) were revealed during the investigation and justice was incomplete. But in the end, I did what I had to do. I told the truth. It wasn't the threats of time at Leavenworth that influenced me as much as the values placed in me during my upbringing. The moment the words left my lips, I sealed both our fates. In my sleep, my interrogator's angry, red face loomed before me, taunting and goading me into a confession. I had loved the Corps. Now, I felt like an outcast, no longer fit for duty ... or life. I had brought shame to the Corps and shame to the man I loved.

That is when I started my periodic descents into the black pit of hell called depression. It is often debated whether traumatic events and the turbulent emotions they spawn contribute to chemical imbalances or neurological dysfunction in the brain or whether depression would happen at some point in time anyway. I may never know for sure, but I believe it likely that these events unleashed the demon that lay dormant, like a cancer, in my mind.

Perhaps that demon was conceived there when I was born, or at the very least, while I was still quite young. It might have begun on the night my brothers and I watched in terror as our father held a loaded pistol to our mom's head in a drunken rage. Or maybe it was on that Christmas night when we stood pajama-clad in the snow with our new toys, waiting for Daddy to make good on his threat to burn the house down. Perhaps it was while I stood on one side of my bedroom door with my mom who was pregnant with my youngest brother, trying to keep my inebriated dad from breaking in.

If it is true that children need some of the same ingredients to grow as plants, chief among them being good "soil," sunlight and water, then you could say I grew up in a family whose soil needed more than a little fertilizing. We had our share of black, stormy days as well as sunny ones. We were a dysfunctional family, to say the least, considering my father was a mentally ill alcoholic, prone to violence during his drinking bouts.

The soil, then, is our parentage, something over which we have no control. Sunlight and water are quite literally necessary for our health. But an old Scotsman, a born philosopher, explained it like this: "The human spirit perishes without the sun; that is why you find so many neurotics in northern climates. I once sailed on a vessel for three weeks and did not see a crack in the clouds. The crew became morose and gloomy and sick. But I had a secret that kept me up. Every day I would go out when the clouds hung low and do two things. One, I remembered the golden sunlight of days past, and two, I thought of the golden sunlight that would come when those clouds had rolled away. Thus, I made my own sunlight. I distilled it in my heart, I manufactured it in my mind."[2] Those words represent a key premise in recovery strategy for the depressed person.

To a child, it can be difficult to manufacture a sunny disposition when you live in a world where storms blow up suddenly and without warning. Later, as an adult, you tend to forget about the sun. But it's still there.

The term "dysfunctional" is almost becoming trite these days. One therapist I saw for awhile went so far as to suggest that all families are dysfunctional to some degree. When viewed on a scale of dysfunctional to perfect, I suppose most families would fall closer to the former end of the scale. I don't agree with my therapist's rationale completely, however. I am an eternal optimist. The term dysfunctional had to be invented to show that something was out of kilter. While there are no perfect families, there are many families that work rather well and produce successful, well-adjusted offspring. There are unquestionably fewer of these families around today than there were in my parents' generation, but they are still there.

I was blessed with the opportunity to associate with one such family during my college years. They were a wonderful, Christian family with two daughters and a son. One daughter was a little younger, the other a little older than I, and we all attended college together where their father headed the campus dairy. The Osingas were an Old World Dutch family. Probably the most significant lesson I cherish from them came through their chastisement when they heard me say the words "I could have or should have. ..." They were very positive, forward-looking people who had lived through the Nazi occupation of Holland. What they were teaching me was to live my life in such a way as to avoid looking back with regrets. Many times when I have felt tempted to speak those words over the years, I've stopped short, remembering their injunction. I suppose I didn't hear the Osinga's message enough. Lessons seem to take better when they're taught in your own home.

While I have seen figures attempting to substantiate that the traditional, nuclear family is nearly extinct, I tend to put more stock in the results of a study conducted in recent years by the National Commission on America's Urban Families stating that more than 57 percent of American families consist of two parents dwelling under the same roof.[3] One would logically assume that healthy individuals are more likely to be reared in these homes than in broken homes. Of course, dwelling under the same roof doesn't necessarily define a healthy family. Parenting is a tough, full-time job, but too many parents are abdicating this responsibility to schools, neighbors and the media — the so-called village. Many American children are growing up with warped values as a result of the entertainment/information media which baby-sit them — television, movies, music, video games and the Internet. Kids who should be at home with a parent or other family member are more often found in malls or on the streets, seeking approval from other misguided juveniles or adults. On the outside, these families seem normal. Many live in quiet suburbs. They drive nice cars, take great vacations, have stylish clothes and never go hungry. Yet, all too often there is a deep, spiritual hunger and emotional vacuum in their lives.

No matter what kind of job our parents did raising us, we can't spend our adult lives blaming them for our problems. I did try to do that for a while in young adulthood. It was easy to blame my father, whose paternal influence and visible love were sadly missing in my childhood. I even blamed my mother, whose love and approval I felt as if I had to earn, probably due more to her preoccupation with my father's illness than to any real negligence on her part. I grew up feeling alienated from both my parents to some degree.

Thankfully, I was never physically abused, to my conscious recollection, but I was molested by a 16-year-old cousin when I was eight, which I tried for much of my life to forget. It took me a long time to even bring that event up in counseling because I'd always thought I was somehow responsible for it — not a very healthy thought to carry into adolescence or adulthood. Still, my basic needs were provided for. I was loved and, essentially, I was nurtured. My mother insured that my brothers and I were raised in the Christian tradition. I unfortunately received mixed signals from my parents in the form of intermittent encouragement and criticism. Consequently, I intermittently both believed in myself and doubted my abilities.

I can say, without fear of retribution from either parent, that I received some inadvertent emotional abuse as a child. Any child raised in a home with warring parents is emotionally scarred. I joke with my mother today about the 12 perfect school attendance certificates I received, which attest to the fact that I was never allowed to stay home, no matter how sick I thought I might have been. I missed the occasional morning or afternoon, just enough to keep my infernal record intact. And yes, Mom, I did start a German measles epidemic in fourth grade! But, I was blessed with unusually good health, I must admit — that and the ability to get sick on weekends and holidays. Whether I was influenced by a perfectionistic mother or I was just bent that way myself, I had a lot of self-discipline as a child. I tried once to catch mumps from my brother because

I wanted to stay home and be babied so much! Eventually, I just expected myself to stay healthy. I became intolerant of mistakes, both my own and those of others. People like me no doubt gravitate toward military service for good reason.

While we have no choice but to give credit, at least in part, for our emotional development to our parents, we do have some choice when we reach an age of responsibility with regard to how much we will let our emotions rule us. Clinical depression is recognized today as an emotional state of debilitating sadness and withdrawal, represented by a faulty balance of certain critical chemicals in the brain, or possibly by structural changes in the brain. It is a condition that can be genetic. Environmental factors can also induce some serious forms of depression. When our brain chemistry is normal, we are generally equipped to handle life's ups and downs. We still have the ability to remember the sunshine. When we are chemically unbalanced, we need specialized help. There is still a sort of chicken-and-egg debate as to whether a pre-existing chemical imbalance or structural anomaly causes depression or whether depression simply manifests itself chemically or otherwise in our brains. There are really two major facets of depression: the psychological-spiritual and the biological-physical.

My family history certainly bears out the gene theory. Recent research has shed much light on the supposed genetic properties of depression. But there are also some pervasive psycho-social factors in my extended family than span several generations. It is the question of choice that is open to so much speculation, both by the medical community and by those of us who have experienced severe, protracted depression. To what extent can we unlearn what we have learned in experiencing emotional or mental illness? To what extent are we simply at the apparent unrelenting mercy of biochemical impulses?

Fortunately, we can deal with both areas. In my own case, that's what I did. While I received various types of therapy for years dealing with the psychodynamic roots of my depression, it took treating my assumed chemical imbalance with drug therapy in order for me to truly begin recovering. After the depressive episodes subsided, I could focus more effectively on the issues I had been grappling with for much of my life. In a depressive crisis, we may need mental "first aid." True healing is a longer process. Still, some people suffering from severe depression will not require drug therapy while others appear to recover with antidepressant medication and very little psychotherapy. Effective treatments vary depending on the length and severity of the depression and on its root causes. Even mild or moderate depression can be debilitating and should not be taken lightly.

The doctor whose observations and treatment ultimately led me to recovery termed my case a 60-40 case: nonfunctionally depressed about 60 percent of the time, functionally normal about 40 percent of the time. I suffered from severe, recurrent Major Depressive Disorder (MDD) that was worsening as time went on. No one who knew me intimately in those days would dispute that.

I had been raised with a deep sense of conscience, which led to inner conflict over the fluid value system I began acquiring in my college years during the "liberating" and self-centered '70s. I was aware I had made mistakes and I badly wanted to rectify them. I felt rather isolated from the rest of the world during the public unraveling of my first marriage. Turning back to my roots of Christianity for the answers I so desperately needed, I gained some inner peace over time. But despite all that, I still could not escape the throes of debilitating depression. It wasn't making sense. To my thinking, a repentant spirit and time should have begun to heal me, but it wasn't happening. My problems were much deeper than I realized. Thus began my quest for true healing.

I don't believe anyone who is depressed actually wants to be in that state of mind. There are those who have postulated over the years that depression is a learned means of escape from reality or responsibility. Of that, I am unsure. But I do believe that once a person is battling depression, that individual's will to recover will have a significant impact on the outcome. I observed some interesting things during the time I spent in a recovery support group for women suffering from everything from depression to various addictions. While I was sure some of those women were miserable and were there to seek a way out, I was just as sure that some of them were never going to find it. I believe they had acquiesced too much to their condition. These women gave lip service to their desire for recovery, but they didn't really believe they could overcome. I could see it in their eyes, the windows to their souls.

If there is one way in which I differed from most of these women, it is that during my lucid, up times, I refused to stop believing there was a solution somewhere, somehow to my illness. I did my best to keep this hope alive. In the depths of depression, rational thought is almost nonexistent. But faith, which is not a rational, logical concept, can exist. Sometimes I survived on a tiny shred of faith in God, or even faith in other stronger people, that led to just enough hope to get me to the next oasis of relief. But in my worst times, while I was never aware of being overtly suicidal, I remember wanting to die. In fact, I had an irrational fixation on death and often lived in an atmosphere of oppressive foreboding. At times, I wondered if it was just the stubbornness I inherited from my ancestors that kept me going. If I inherited my illness, I also inherited along with it a strong bent toward self-determination. At times it propelled me forward with a relentless drive, but it could also keep me locked up in isolation, trying to "fix" myself without the help of others.

My depression and associated anxiety often manifested itself in lengthy periods — the longest being six weeks — during which I slept and ate little. The hellish hours of nighttime insomnia were the worst times I had to endure. Life slowly drained out of me during those dark bouts with my demons. On several occasions, I nearly lost consciousness because of low blood sugar and exhaustion. It was in the midst of fighting to keep blackness from enveloping me that I realized how much I truly wanted to live. If I gave in, I feared never waking up again. I believe my daughter, Jennifer, might literally have saved my life when she was a toddler. I collapsed getting out of bed one morning, and felt myself drifting away. I was near to letting go of life, so desperately wanting release. But my angel appeared at the doorway just in time for me to focus on her worried, little face. "What's wrong, Mommy?" she asked. "I'll help you." She reached down with her little hand and I felt the strong hands of God lift me off the floor.

I always believed I had been brought into the world for a purpose. No matter how painful, I persevered so that I might discover that purpose. Sometimes, I wondered how different my existence was from that of a prisoner of war. There is no prison more bleak than that of the mind, and depression can be one of the manifestations of spiritual warfare. It wasn't just my perseverance that kept me from giving in. I couldn't possibly have held on to my sanity or my life without the devotion of my husband. Russ was the most crucial member of my support team. In addition, an entire network of family members and friends prayed for me for years. I honestly felt as if God had assigned a special squadron of angels to watch over me. Perhaps He did.

I found that music played an important role in my recovery. I'd been directed to the Psalms by my pastor as a means of providing solace when my soul was troubled. Others had suggested singing songs of praise to lift my spirits. When you're depressed, the last thing you want to do is sing or even listen to uplifting music, but it is one of the best medicines. It has been said that music is a universal language that speaks to the soul. Music therapy is a tool used to "promote healthy psychological responses in patients by decreasing stress and anxiety, facilitating self-expression and creativity and increasing feelings of self-worth," said music therapist Pamela Kaney in *Christian Counseling Today* magazine in 1998. "Music is a powerful tool God has left lying around for anyone to pick up and use," she further stated.[4] Not only did singing or listening to music sometimes lift me up when I felt myself sliding down into the pit of despair, but I learned a good maintenance dose on a regular basis went a long way toward preventing depression. One of my fondest memories of growing up was hearing my mom sing and whistle around the house while doing chores. I'm sure she knew that "a cheerful heart is good medicine,"[5] even though she had a few challenges with depression, herself. Her singing brought a sense of warmth and security to an otherwise insecure household.

Joni Eareckson Tada, a paraplegic from a diving accident as a young teenager, and someone well-acquainted with depression, writes in one of her more recent books, *A Quiet*

Place in a Crazy World:

> Our words of praise reach farther than we can imagine. Victory is found in praise. The outer realms of darkness shudder with the repercussions of our praise, and our words of adoration to the Lord have a rippling effect throughout all of heaven and hell. Devils scatter and strongholds are shattered.[6]

In addition to praise, there were other controllable factors that could contribute to my well-being, such as diet and exercise. Building up my reserves of energy was necessary, since I didn't know when my next "attack" would come. In biochemical warfare, one of the secret weapons we all have are endorphins, which chemically act as the body's natural mood elevators. It is now a well-established fact that we can stimulate the release of endorphins and thus, a sense of well-being, through exercise as simple as walking or through hearty laughter. One of the best-known cases of the remarkable healing quality of endorphins and a positive outlook, in general, is that of Norman Cousins who documented his experiences in his book, *Anatomy of an Illness*. He suffered from a rare, life-threatening collagen disease, which he reversed completely through what many saw as an unorthodox, if not ridiculous laughter therapy. Regardless of how unorthodox it seemed, no one could question its efficacy.

Far more orthodox, perhaps, than watching slapstick comedy or listening to jokes around the clock is a practice we are encouraged to engage in by the Apostle Paul in the New Testament:

> Finally, brothers, whatever is true, whatever is noble, whatever is right, whatever is pure, whatever is lovely, whatever is admirable — if anything is excellent or praiseworthy — think about such things.[7]

Our thoughts and our speech have a great impact on the way we feel and act. Most of us are familiar with the words of

Solomon, "As he thinketh in his heart, so is he."[8] James has a good deal to say about speech in the New Testament, as well. He compares the tongue to the bit in a horse's mouth or the rudder of a ship in its directional power over our lives. Proverbs also tells us, "The tongue has the power of life and death and those who love it will eat its fruit."[9] Likewise, "Reckless words pierce like a sword, but the tongue of the wise brings *healing*."[10] Not only can harm be done by speaking unkindly to others, but we can inflict great injury on ourselves with our own self-talk. Psychologist Shad Helmstetter says in his book, *The Self-talk Solution,* that up to 75 percent of our brain's programming comes from the negative input we have either received from others or given ourselves from birth.[11] This self-talk is both conscious and unconscious. No wonder so many people struggle with depression! Reprogramming our thought processes is known as cognitive restructuring in the psychiatric world. It is highly effective in treating depression and other mental illnesses.

I believe the body and the mind have the innate ability to heal themselves in very similar ways. One of the keys to releasing our natural healing agents is how we think. Dr. Bernie Siegel in his book, *Peace, Love and Healing,* maintains that we all have a sort of sixth sense which activates our healing system. But in order to make it work, we must let go of guilt.[12] That can be a tall order for some people. Guilt is an especially big barrier for those who are depressed. We must believe ourselves worthy of being healed and learn to forgive ourselves for past mistakes. A friend of mine, a former special education teacher, likes to say that we must remember we all have erasers at the end of our pencils. The role of guilt in depression and how it affected me will be discussed in more detail later.

As our state of mind can drastically affect our physical healing processes, it also follows that various actions can affect our mental health. Many times I used a process I called "going through the motions" to begin regaining my mental stability when I was depressed. Though I didn't feel like it, I forced myself to act happy, to seek out people and activities that broke me out of my isolation and inertia. It is a proven fact that jokes are funnier when a person is smiling. *Act* happy and you put into motion a process that will actually make you *feel* happier. Psychologists call this Rational Emotive Therapy (RET), for those of you who like labels. Whether or not it is in vogue anymore is immaterial. It can and does work.

Russ and I for several years participated in a weekly home-based business activity known simply as a Friday Night Session. This consisted of gathering business associates around us for training and motivation. I was compelled to take an up-front role as a teacher, many times when I was miserably depressed. It was definitely going through the motions and nothing more for me during those times. Yet, more often than not, that association pulled me out of my black moods. There is a strong edification process at work in some home-based business organizations. Financial success is not as important to some people as inner growth. Many people just need to have their self-worth validated. Much healing can occur in this kind of atmosphere. Not only do we gain the collective energy and focus that Napoleon Hill called the "mastermind" concept, but when we come together in this type of setting, we are sometimes engaging in an informal type of group therapy. It just proves the old adage that we need each other. A similar process occurs in church home fellowships or Bible study groups and in various support groups. These types of settings can be highly effective in addressing and integrating an array of human needs. There are churches and ministries that do this extremely well, but the biblical laws that govern emotional health and prosperity (a slippery word) are not always clearly delineated from the pulpit.

Norman Cousins in his book, *The Healing Heart*, says we retain control over our illnesses by "recognizing the existence of resources represented by the healing system and the belief system that activates it. And the belief system is not just a collection of mechanical parts but a confluence of values and attitudes — hope, faith, confidence, purpose, will to live and a capacity for joyous living."[13] We naturally strive toward the goal of joyous living, but many of us block our own paths to freedom by holding onto our pain. We all deserve to live joyful lives. Simply making a decision to do so can *start* us on the road to recovery when we suffer from depression. We bear a large part of the responsibility for staying on the road. If Norman Cousins had achieved only a spiritual healing from his famed illness, he would have had something to celebrate, as well — even if his disease had proved fatal. "For what does it profit a man to gain the whole world, and forfeit his soul?"[14]

Did I *choose* to suffer for so long without the aid of antidepressant medication? I truly believed at first I could recover without drugs. I prayed for years for a drug-free healing. I experienced a genuine revulsion to drug therapy because of my father's abuse of alcohol, but perhaps even more so because I had a brother who was a drug abuser. Also, no one even suggested antidepressants for several years. One psychiatrist theorized I suffered from a type of bipolar disorder (formerly called manic-depressive illness) and wanted to treat me with lithium, which I refused to take because of his aggressive manner and hasty diagnosis. This doctor had a rubber stamp approach. At times, my illness bore a resemblance to bipolar disorder, but neither my physician of choice nor I believe that was the correct diagnosis. (Bipolar disorder, in layman's terms, is a form of mental illness characterized by severe moods swings from depression to mania or a highly stimulated state of mind in which a person may be hyperactive and restless, feeling unlimited energy or clarity of thought. This illness has several classifications).

After my illness resulted in my losing two jobs from repeated absenteeism, I decided to stay at home and concentrate on my health. Without the pressures of full-time employment, or children, who had not come along yet, I experienced a remission period of two years. I thought I had, indeed, recovered permanently. It was three months after the birth of our first child that I relapsed into severe, postpartum depression. Three months after that, I discovered I was pregnant again. From then on, the pressures of motherhood (to say nothing of hormone imbalances), coupled with the guilt my illness compelled me to feel, both hastened and lengthened my bouts of depression.

Following the birth of our second daughter, I was prescribed an antidepressant which I refused because I didn't trust the doctor who prescribed it. I had to be convinced beyond the shadow of a doubt that medication was necessary. Another factor contributing to my fear of drugs was that I had observed an uncle's wife who suffered from clinical depression appear robot-like while medicated, and I couldn't bear the thought of becoming that way. It wasn't until I came to the point where I had no more options that I agreed to try antidepressants. This time, I decided to trust my doctor completely, and that enhanced my treatment, I'm sure. He specialized in pharmacology and was able to alleviate my fears. I continued in drug therapy for five years, and I was anything but a robot. It had taken me 10 years of suffering from depression before I was able to receive an accurate and complete diagnosis. No one should have to suffer that long. Some suffer much longer. Fortunately, more information on treatment options is available to the general public today.

By the time I began my treatment, I had been pruned nearly to the roots. I petitioned God many times for the answer to why I had been allowed to experience all this. I thought of the Apostle Paul in the New Testament and his "thorn in the flesh." God never gave me an answer any different from the one He gave His saint: "My grace is sufficient for you, for my power is made perfect in weakness."[15] I read accounts of great leaders who had suffered from my affliction (Winston Churchill, Abraham Lincoln, Charles Spurgeon and Martin Luther are among them). Surely God had used them for greatness, despite their affliction. I began to vow that I would seek ways to serve God, and my fellow man, regardless of whether I had to accept my condition with grace or whether He chose to heal me.

Today, nearly seven years off all medication, I can say with confidence I am healed. I have not forgotten my vow. I feel I have no choice but to minister to other souls facing their own private hells and to give them the message of hope. That is why I write this book and why I publicly and privately share my healing experience when I have the opportunity.

Two

One isn't born oneself. One is born with a mass of expectations, a mass of other people's ideas — and you have to work through it all.

V.S. Naipaul

~~~~~~~~~~~~

My Parents' Child

People who suffer from depression do not exist in a vacuum. They are someone's children, someone's brothers or sisters and maybe even parents, themselves. From the moment of birth and arguably, from the moment of conception, we all began a relationship with our parents. The temperaments we have are a gift from God more than the result of parental influence. He endowed us each with a unique personality that would incline us to be "bent" in a certain way. Wise is the parent who discovers how a child is bent and seeks to help the child to develop positively in that direction, within the confines of wisdom and moral law. Unfortunate is the child (and the parent) who has to endure an upbringing of being molded as a selfish parent wishes him or her to be.

Parent-child relationships range from the ideal loving, nurturing, limit-setting bond all the way to the opposite extreme of indifference, abandonment or even outright abuse. Sadly, there is a vast sea of families who fall into an array of categories between the two extremes. Educators and Sunday School teachers encounter many bruised children on a regular basis. They give themselves away by exhibiting excessive neediness in one way or another. There are others (I was one of them) who are so quiet and well-behaved, they often become "teachers' pets."

Approval-seeking is another form of neediness exhibited by a child who may get little approval at home. This is not to say that all quiet, well-behaved children have hidden problems. I merely point out that those who do often get overlooked until it is too late to take early corrective action.

Old-fashioned common sense goes a long way toward uncovering emotional problems. I have already established that my family life as a child was far from ideal, though my very early recollections were of a seemingly normal, happy home life. These were the days before alcohol began to consume my father. I came along when my parents were still fairly young. My mother was 21 and my father was 25. My three brothers and I (I am the second-born) are all Baby Boomers. We were born into a world that forced us to deal with the harsh realities of competition and the technical revolution. I remember feeling as if I coexisted in two worlds — the more gentile world of my parents that fixed many of my values, and the burgeoning "new" world that could leave me feeling so insignificant and out of place.

My father was a self-employed building contractor who had a thriving business. My mother wanted nothing more than to be a homemaker, occasionally helping my father with bookkeeping. She had been offered a home economics scholarship to college, but turned it down, even though she was valedictorian of her high school class. She had planned to be an interior decorator. My parents had eloped to marry when they were 16 and 19 years old, respectively. Mom had two miscarriages before she gave birth to my brother at the age of 18. She was more mature than most young women, which was both a blessing and a curse from my point of view as the only daughter who later had to follow in her footsteps. But perhaps she had tried to grow up too fast. Some time after my older brother was born, for reasons she has only partially revealed, my mom attempted suicide.

I am at least the fourth generation manifesting depression on my mother's side, and my father's family tree looks similar. There has been depression on my husband's family tree, as well. Of course, I would like to see the buck stop here, with me, but I know everyone from here on must walk his or her life's path. They will face challenges and makes choices, and I won't always be there to intervene. I can't play God. I am not fearful that my daughters have "the dreaded gene." They live in a home environment far more nurturing and positive than the one I grew up in, and that carries a lot of weight.

To this day, I value many of the examples my mother set for me. Her moral values were unquestioned. I know she wanted nothing but the best for her children. She had high standards, and she expected that her children would adopt those standards. As the only daughter in the family, I felt she was particularly watchful over me. I recall feeling so much pressure to excel academically and in my homemaking skills that I once made the comment to her that I just wanted to be average. You can imagine what kind of reaction that evoked from my mom!

When I reached my predictably rebellious teenage years, my mother and I battled constantly over my priorities. I felt she was trying to recapture some of her lost youth vicariously through me. She felt I was disrespectful of her wishes. She is very old-school when it comes to absolute parental authority. In retrospect, we were both right and wrong. It wasn't the idea of authority I resented, it was her method of communication. Whether she liked it or not, I was as headstrong as she. (This trait has been passed to the next generation, and I'm poised for potential conflict with my own daughters. I call this stage "parenting college"). The battleground was set for more conflict and more rebellion on my part. Actually, our arguments were mostly a tool for venting our private anger and woundedness, which was not necessarily toward each other. This made the conflict even more unhealthy. I would have benefited, no doubt, from being on my high school debate team but for one problem: Mom was the coach. I did give serious thought in college to becoming a lawyer. It's likely I'd have been a vicious one, but I was afraid of public speaking. Instead I learned to use writing as an emotional steam vent.

To the casual observer, nothing seemed amiss in my relationship with my mother. I haven't analyzed other mother-daughter relationships in a clinical sort of way. I'm sure I compared notes with my friends, as most young folks do. We just couldn't seem to get emotionally close. I was thought of almost universally (my mother appearing at the time to be the exception) as a polite, well-behaved daughter. It felt good to have the occasional confirmation by a teacher or other adult of my self-worth. And lest I be accused of mother-bashing, let me add that I learned much later in life just how highly my mom valued me. I wish she had been able to express those feelings more often, but when we weren't too busy having shouting matches, she was dealing with the pain of my dad's problems. All this set the stage in my home for conflict and criticism rather than praise.

I never truly believed that Mom didn't love me. I knew she did. But her terms and mine were different. In providing all my basic needs, my mom was unexcelled. She went to great lengths to do some special things for me, such as sewing beautiful clothes for years. I still have the formal dress she made for my first high school prom. She worked on it into the wee hours the day of the dance, despite having a migraine headache. Whenever I look at it, I remember the love that went into making it. She saw to it that we had a piano when we couldn't really afford one just so I could take music lessons. She bought me a clarinet and let me join the school band when I grew tired of the piano because my best friend was playing the clarinet. That was love in action. Because I knew that, even when I was young, it seemed petty and immature to think harshly of my mom for any of her shortcomings. Who knows how my own daughters may relate to me as teenagers or young adults?

Despite my early feelings of being misunderstood and alienated from my mother, we have a much closer relationship today. It isn't perfect. We naïvely thought we could dwell under the same roof for a while when Russ and I relocated our family to Virginia last year. It wasn't long before old wounds started throbbing, but I believe each of us has come to respect the other's viewpoint. I remember crying out for Mom inwardly in the middle of an exhaustive night while rocking a sick baby. I'm sure I could not feel the kind of love and nurturing I feel for my children today had I not experienced the same from her. In fact, I feel I must have been exceptionally loved in my earliest years. I believe that is where my great capacity for love and empathy had its origins. I also believe my emotional development may have been short-circuited somewhere in my early years because of my mom's occasional battles with depression and her difficulty in connecting emotionally. We never really had an opportunity to get back on track because of the upheaval that my dad's alcohol problems brought to our lives.

I have tried to recall specific memories of tender, nurturing moments with my mom. I only have a few. The injustice to my mom is that in repressing painful memories, I let some of the good go with the bad. One of those memories I'm glad I held onto is the way she used to wake me in the morning by sitting on the side of the bed and rubbing my back, often singing a little song. I continued that tradition with my own daughters. It helped me to reconnect with my childhood. I know my mom did the best she could, and I made the choice a long time ago to love her for it. I hope she understands how frequently emotional wounds can occur in any family. In most cases, they are never intended. I'm just thankful they can be healed.

My earlier relationship with my father was a very tenuous one. More often than not, he was not around. He was either off in Florida on fishing trips with his drinking buddies or sitting in his favorite tavern until the wee hours or in a mental institution. I have very few sketchy memories of him in any semblance of a family setting. I treasure those few memories I do have. We vacationed together as a family several times when I was young. Those times I remember as being marred by my father's drunken fits. There was a lot of yelling, cursing and verbal abuse of my mother when he was drinking. We lived in a state of fear and uncertainty. Usually, his bark was worse than his bite, but there were some violent outbursts during which we children (I had two brothers then, and later, a third) feared that Mom would be hurt. The worst occurred on that night when we witnessed Daddy grab Mom and hold the pistol to her head. She looked him in the eye and dared him to pull the trigger. We hastily plotted to overtake him with baseball bats and kill him if we had to. I honestly believe we might have had he not backed down. I remember waking in the middle of the night on more than one occasion in the car going to our grandparents' house where Mom would take us for safety until Daddy could sober up.

My dad lost his business and my mom was forced to go back to school and become a teacher. She sold encyclopedia sets on the side to help make ends meet. She refused to give up on Daddy for a long time, but finally felt her only option left was to seek a divorce when I was 15. We lived through times of being all but destitute and could not have survived had it not been for my grandparents. I think I started hating my father when he had our social security benefits terminated. I saw that as mean-spirited. My mother has shared with me in recent years that several times she had despairing thoughts of ending all our lives during those awful times. God must have intervened with just a little more hope when she needed it. She never shrank from her responsibility. Though I must have inherited some of the genes that governed my temperament from my mom (a melancholy-sanguine combination), I'm glad her mental toughness exceeded mine. Otherwise, I may not be here today. Had I been in her shoes in those circumstances, I might have succumbed to the pressures of life.

Despite the fact that we were not a whole family, our home was a Christian home. We were in church nearly every Sunday. Mom was deeply involved in the church, and we kids were in all sorts of church and other activities. It was the only real stability in our lives, besides my grandparents. The people in our church were good, solid, salt-of-the-earth neighbors. From time to time, folks would greet Mom with a friendly handshake and press a $20 bill or whatever they could afford into her hand. There was a strong sense of community and helping those in need. It was a way of life. We never forgot their generosity. I remember Mom passing along whatever charity she could to those less fortunate than we were. She donated clothing and food to indigent families. Through the church, she organized Christmas-in-July baskets for the needy. I remember helping her fill them and wrap them with brightly colored cellophane.

To this day, I have heart-felt gratitude for the love and caring my grandparents provided to my brothers and me. They were like a second set of parents to us. In fact, we still call our grandmother "Mother" the same as her own children do. Growing up with an extended family, which also included aunts and uncles, was a privilege that many children, including my own until this year, don't enjoy in this era. I have wonderful memory upon memory of special events with my grandparents. Going to visit Mother and Papa Shock was one of the highlights of our childhood. They still lived in the old family farmhouse on 100 prime Virginia acres where most all their children were born until I was about five years old. The farm was a magical place of adventure with an abundance of secret hideouts to explore. Even going with my grandmother to the well or the spring to draw up a bucket of water was an adventure. Not so enjoyable, but unavoidable, were those scary trips to the outhouse!

My dad built a new home (with indoor plumbing) for my grandparents on a rolling, five-acre parcel surrounded by scenic Blue Ridge mountain vistas just up the road from the old farm, which was sold during lean times. It was here that many wonderful childhood memories had their origins. My heart still quickens when I drive those old, country roads and see the nearby mountains. Among the best memories were the Sunday and holiday meals we shared around the big family table, topped off by one of Mother's wonderful deserts. She baked the best cakes and pies I ever tasted. I can still hear my grandfather, who died in 1993, spinning yarns from the Great Depression era. And how well I remember and appreciate today the many times I sat at the kitchen table and listened to Papa Shock read the Bible and pray during family devotions or expound on politics. Every year as Father's Day approaches, I recall with great affection how devoted my grandfather was to my grandmother and, likewise, to his entire family. I can still see him standing in the kitchen, smiling and peeling potatoes or making a salad for supper, about the only mealtime chore Mother would allow him to have, but one he did lovingly.

I miss those days when food was more than measurable grams of fat or protein. It was just plain good — good for the body and the soul. More than the food itself, it was the way we partook of it — long, leisurely meals surrounded by family — that made it special. Then we all got too educated, and too busy. Papa Shock believed that when you were ailing, you just needed to eat something. He took sustenance for headaches or stomach aches or whatever aches came along. I don't believe that man was ever depressed a day in his life. I'm glad his blood courses through my veins. I am ever so thankful for the strong, fatherly influence he had on my life. My grandparents were my anchor during the turbulent times of my childhood, and today I can still comfort myself with a little Southern soul food when I'm feeling a bit down.

The woods behind my grandparents' house seemed almost enchanted when I was a child. My brothers and I spent many an hour exploring and swinging on grapevines. I learned to play a pretty fair game of eight ball on their old-fashioned pool table. More often than not, I was "one of the guys," playing touch football with my brothers in the yard or shooting hoops on the basketball goal nailed onto an old pine tree. When I needed a quieter moment to myself, I sat in the rocking chair in the solitude of the living room and read *Guideposts* or *HomeLife* or thumbed through old yearbooks from my aunt's and uncles' school days.

On other occasions, I simply got alone with nature, walking off into the woods by myself to marvel at the beauty of God's creation. This has been a lifelong habit with me. I have always gained some serenity and the ability to see things more clearly while in the outdoors, especially if there's a mountain in view. I will forever be grateful for my country upbringing. I love what Anne Frank, whose insight and strength we know from her diary during her days of hiding to escape Nazi imprisonment and persecution, said about nature's sedative effect:

> The best remedy for those who are afraid, lonely or unhappy is to go outside, somewhere where they can be quite alone with the heavens, nature, and God. Because only then does one feel that all is as it should be and that God wishes to see people happy, amidst the simple beauty of nature. As long as this exists, and it certainly always will, I know that then there will always be comfort for every sorrow, whatever the circumstances may be.[1]

I don't know if young Anne was acquainted with the writings of Henry David Thoreau, but I'm sure they could have found much about which to agree. Thoreau was also a lover of nature, and writes simply but eloquently in his essay entitled "Walking" about the art of sauntering, a term which was most probably derived from the Middle Ages pilgrims who were always on their way `*a la Sainte Terre* — to the Holy Land. As Thoreau says, "For every walk is a sort of crusade, preached by some Peter the Hermit in us, to go forth and reconquer this Holy Land from the hands of the Infidels."[2]

I'm not sure if I knew when I was young exactly who the infidels were, but I'm certain they didn't live next door to us, for that residence was our church parsonage, which my dad built. We became close friends of the pastor and his family. Reverend Woodrow Wilson Crady, a man who grew up in Knob Creek, Kentucky where little Abe Lincoln once lived, was always willing to witness in his gentle, loving way to my dad, though it seemed to fall mostly on deaf ears. Having those wonderful people just a cow pasture away from us was a great source of comfort. We romped and played in creeks, in the river and all over fields and hills with the Crady children. I vividly remember one dark night running and stumbling as fast as I could through the large field that separated our houses to alert the Cradys that Daddy was on the rampage again. I'm sure I did that more than once. Our dear pastor had a way of calming him down.

Daddy built the Piney River Baptist Church building, also. Despite the labors of his hands, he did little in a spiritual sense to build the church, rarely, if ever putting in an appearance there. Sunday memories bring a mixture of images: Mom, my brothers and I dressed up and heading off for church and Dad in a tee shirt and jeans sitting in front of the television with a six-pack of beer. I recall the day during the JFK-assassination era we came home from church to learn that Jack Ruby had shot and killed Lee Harvey Oswald, an event Daddy had witnessed live on television. The only pleasant memories I have of Daddy and television are those Saturday nights he and I would sometimes watch boxing together, a sport I learned to appreciate solely to get close to him.

I have memories of early spring afternoons, riding my bike with little patches of snow still on the ground, watching Daddy burn off the garden to prepare it for spring planting. I used to enjoy watching him build things. I admired his strong physique. His strength gave me both a sense of security and fear in his presence. I saw him as potentially life-giving and life-taking. He quite literally saved my mom and all of us kids from a potential fiery death once on a late fall afternoon along the Blue Ridge Parkway when our car engine caught fire. He was able to extinguish it with quick thinking. We were surrounded by miles of dry leaves that one spark would have ignited, to say nothing of the danger of an explosion. This scene strikes a contrasting chord to the snowy Christmas when Daddy was threatening to burn down the house.

There were other Christmases of hiking up into the hills with Daddy to bring home a tree and afterward stopping off at the "Frog Pond" to go ice skating. I still clearly remember Daddy letting my brothers and me sit in his lap and drive my grandfather Hebron's old Model A Ford around the fields. These are times a child never forgets.

My brothers and I took a camping excursion with Daddy one year when fishing season opened. He helped me catch my first fish. He probably drank a little, but he didn't get drunk. (I was moved to tears a decade ago when our older daughter caught her first fish with her dad). There are sketchy memories of a wonderful fishing trip on the Chesapeake Bay, a vacation to the Great Smoky Mountains and a visit to the Outer Banks of North Carolina. For the briefest moments, we mimicked a normal, happy family and life seemed good. I'm grateful for those memories. Fortunately, my dad captured many of them in slides and home movies. They give an ironic permanence to the fleeting moments of happiness we shared.

I longed for my dad to be a part of my activities as I was growing up. Only once, when I was 13 years old, can I remember him watching one of my church-league softball games. I managed to hit a triple down the first base line that day. More exciting than the hit for me was the fact that I could hear my dad cheering and urging me on as I ran the bases. It was one of the happiest memories of my youth. I watched Daddy build with his own hands a beautiful cabin cruiser named the *Debbie Lou,* for me. I proudly told all my friends about "my" boat and invited them to sail on it. My brother got to go along on its launching. That was its only voyage because my dad lapsed into a severe battle with the bottle and ended up selling the boat before I could ride on it. He tried to build another, but couldn't finish. It sat in our yard, half-built until the wood started to decay. I used to sit in it and cry inwardly. I perfected the art of tearless crying.

I was blessed to have my grandfather and several uncles who could fill that fatherly role on occasion. But I think it was my older brother, Harold, who had the greatest paternal, or at least male influence on my life. I truly admired my big brother. He was protective and set the kind of example I wanted to emulate. He was always in pursuit of excellence. I even took on some of his interests, including athletics and sports writing. We both pursued military careers, mine, obviously being cut short. During my lowest times at Camp Lejeune while the threads of my personal life unraveled for all to see, it was Harold and his wife, Donna, who stayed in contact with me and kept me sane. Even though we lived thousands of miles apart for much of our adult lives, we've had a unique emotional bond. When we need to talk, we can really connect. Donna is like a sister to me. Now we live five minutes away from each other.

Still, being the only daughter, I had a special need to be close to my father. I secretly envied my friends who had loving fathers to take them to father-daughter banquets or give them a warm, fatherly embrace. I grew up feeling more unattractive and unworthy than I should have. The need to attach myself to someone led to my premature, ill-fated marriage and other immature relationships. As I approached my college graduation, I longed for my dad to be there to share it with me. After many years of abusing alcohol, he was trying to turn his life around. My older brother had taken a step toward reconciliation with Daddy by undertaking a small construction project with him. Daddy had done well for a while, but had fallen off the wagon. Harold was disillusioned, but I became determined to reach out and let our father know that I had faith in him. Against my mother's wishes, he did come to my graduation. I've never regretted that decision. It was one of only two times Daddy got to see any of his children in cap and gown.

A few months later, Mom, my two younger brothers and I went to Europe where Mom was embarking on what would come to be an 18-year teaching career. While there, I took a position as a governess with an Austrian family and began a correspondence with my dad. It seemed we could appreciate each other more, being so far away from one another. He was just getting involved with Alcoholics Anonymous, and reported to me each milestone of sobriety he was achieving. I rejoiced with him and let him know how proud I was of his courage. He slowly allowed God into his life. He went back to work as a carpenter at a state institution for the mentally disabled and is now semi-retired, living in beautiful central Virginia in a cabin he built out of historic, recycled timbers, next to his boyhood home. A highlight of my recent return home to Virginia was attending a homecoming at that country church Daddy built, at his invitation. I hugged many relatives and old friends that day. We walked around the church, reliving old memories here and there. Later we gathered around the family stained-glass window for a commemorative photograph, which I will cherish.

It was gratifying to see relationships beginning to be restored between Daddy and all of his children. One of the most precious times of my life occurred in 1991 when Russ and I celebrated our 10th wedding anniversary. For some time, I had hoped to celebrate with a traditional wedding ceremony, reaffirming our wedding vows. I had wanted to have as many family members as possible come and attend, but most importantly, all our parents. It had been my long-standing dream for my dad to walk me down the aisle and give me away to the man I loved. Russ and I had been married in a small, outdoor ceremony with only a handful of friends present. Our parents had never even met each other. We lived in California, my parents were in Virginia and Russ' were in Utah. It took a lot of planning, not to mention expense, but it was worth every penny! My dad looked handsome and distinguished in his tuxedo. Everyone got along beautifully. Before the week was over, Russ' stepfather and my dad were planning to visit each other for a fishing trip.

It was our dear friend and pastor, Rick Savage, who first pointed out to me how painful memories could be healed and relationships restored through God's help. He guided me through many prayers of healing and restoration during my dark days. He taught me how to love myself and to acknowledge my feelings. Most importantly, he taught me about the power of forgiveness. It took years of persistence for me to break down the barrier of hatred bred by an unforgiving spirit I had put up between my father and myself, and to some extent, between my mother and myself. I had begun the steps toward reconciliation with Daddy years earlier, but my anniversary project was the last important step in achieving the healing both he and I craved. That ceremony was quite moving because, as the officiating minister, Rick was able to beautifully convey the miracles that had taken place in several lives.

How I wish my grandparents could have shared that day with us! They did, to the extent that video technology was able to convey it. Perhaps it was more fitting that on that day, my dad be the only father figure I really needed. Less than two years later, we lost Papa Shock. God granted me the privilege of communicating my love for him in a special way during the final days of his life in February 1993. As he lay comatose in a hospital bed, his big, strong heart beginning to falter, my mom asked me to sing "Precious Memories" to him one last time. (I had sung that song at his and Mother's 60th wedding anniversary celebration a year earlier). Papa Shock had a grand, tenor voice and this was his favorite song. As I looked into his face and began to sing in the most loving voice I could muster, his eyes flickered open and followed every movement of my lips. He even began mouthing the words with me, though his voice was no longer there! It was a moment I will always treasure. I considered our "duet" a fitting good-bye to my hero, our patriarch. When I think of the word father, his is the image that first comes to mind.

I cannot boast of such golden moments (yet) with my father, but I am hopeful. I am blessed to still have him and the hope of continued reconciliation and bonding in his latter years. I've tried very hard to focus on his good qualities and the particular strengths of character for which I feel I can still honor him as I recall our years together on this earth as father and daughter. Yes, he is flawed, but so am I. I love him and pray for God's wisdom and strength to grow in him. I know my dad has always loved me. He didn't know how to show it during all those years he was a slave to alcohol. I think my dad and I are both taking great delight in seeing each other frequently now that we are living only a short distance away. We're doing our best to recover lost time.

Two Thanksgivings ago my dad called me and gave me a wonderful gift: his honesty. Never before had we talked so openly about the past and about our respective illnesses. It was truly an answer to prayer. This man has probably done more soul-searching than most. Despite the past, he is at peace. I owe a lot of my self-determination to him. Few men would have had the courage to battle back from utter alienation as he did. We share a common bond as veterans of the same war. It includes the exhilaration of winning, even though we came back wounded. It also includes the pain of knowing one of our own, a son and a brother, may never come back. Greg, the brother just younger than I, has battled depression and substance-abuse psychosis for many years. He hasn't been able to get off the battlefield. Nor has any of us been able to rescue him.

There are few realizations as agonizing as that of reaching out to a loved one who can't or won't reach back. Yes, I know the chasm that often exists between the mentally ill and their families. I also know there is but one unshakable bridge: the cross upon which Jesus Christ died. Those who choose to walk across that bridge leave behind the land of death and of sorrows and enter the land of the joyful living. It can and does happen. For loved ones who don't recover, whose damaged mental capacities may fall short of understanding, there is the hope that God reserves a final place of illumination for them. This I pray for my brother, with a heart full of love and empathy.

Three

No matter how good things get, my capacity to make myself unhappy is always equal to it.

Hugh Prather

~~~~~~~~~~~~

The Anatomy Of Depression

When I mentioned to an acquaintance of mine early in this undertaking that I was writing a book about depression and that I had recovered several years earlier, I was somewhat surprised when she took me aside and said she needed to talk with me about some problems she was having. "What are the symptoms you had?" she wanted to know. I learned that she had felt somewhat driven to be involved in many activities, but was having difficulty coping with all the stress and was having some symptoms of depression. In short, she was overwhelmed and it was leading her to withdraw, much to her husband's concern. She was wondering if she should seek counseling or treatment. My first thought was to suggest that she lighten her load.

I don't pretend to be a doctor, so the best advice I can give to someone who is feeling depressed to any degree is to visit your family doctor to discuss your problems. Sometimes, there can be underlying physical causes to feelings such as those my friend described. Depression is not uncommon, so many doctors can recognize it right away. I don't believe we need to be pressured into seeking out and exorcising our demons at this stage. A thorough and practical examination is the best approach when suspecting that you have symptoms of depression, whether it be a mild or more serious form. As the expression goes, it doesn't take a rocket scientist to figure out you're depressed. But self-treating is not necessarily advisable.

How do you know what to look for? There are some universally accepted symptoms of depression, and a general practitioner may be the first stop in determining whether these symptoms are related to a physiological or a psychological problem. Incidentally, not all physicians are equally qualified to treat depression. Recognizing it is one thing; treating it is another. Serious depression may be best diagnosed and treated, at least initially, by a psychiatrist or a psychologist who can prescribe medication, unless you're fortunate enough to have a family physician who is experienced in dealing with depressed patients. Homeopathy, a much older and natural form of medicine, is another course of treatment you can pursue.

The National Institute of Mental Health (NIMH) recognizes 10 symptoms of depression. Anyone who experiences as many as five of these symptoms listed below for more than two weeks, says the NIMH, may have a depressive illness that requires treatment:

1. Persistent low or anxious feelings
2. Decreased energy
3. Loss of interest in usual activities; loss of sex drive
4. Sleep disturbances
5. Appetite and weight changes
6. Feelings of hopelessness
7. Feelings of guilt or worthlessness
8. Thoughts of death or suicide
9. Difficulty in concentrating or making decisions
10. Chronic aches or physical discomfort[1]

I had all the above, and then some. My depression was episodic, progressing to chronic proportions in its latter stages.

What causes depression? There are several classic theories, but research is shedding more and more light on depression and other affective disorders. Of course, we've come a long way since the days of Hippocrates or since Robert Burton, the 17th-century scholar, penned his famous book, *Anatomy of Melancholy*, in which he offered some curiously accurate theories of depression's causes, as well as some amusingly inaccurate ones. (Ironically and prophetically, I acquired an old, worn copy of that book from my college librarian while I was still attending school, before the onset of my illness). For the sake of the broader discussion, some of the historical theories need to be mentioned. Repressed anger is the accepted psychoanalytic theory of what causes depression. According to Frank Bruno, Ph.D. in his book, *Psychological Symptoms*, depressed people, in Freudian terms, "have super-egos that are overly strict and self-punitive. (The superego is the moral agent of the personality). Consequently, they have a hard time expressing normal aggressive feelings in the face of life's many frustrations. They bottle up their hostile feelings, and this gets converted into depression."[2]

These types of closed, secretly hostile attitudes have been shown to be influential factors in the onset of other crippling diseases. Bernie Siegel has pointed out that "a stoic, self-denying personality is the most commonly cited psychological factor in the development of cancer."[3] The NIMH reported in a 1996 study a link between stress hormones, depression and cancer. *Psychology Today* reported in August 1997 and again in April 1999 that people who have had a major episode of depression also are far more likely to develop heart disease.[4] So is the answer for these people to let it all out? Just blow up and feel better? It's not that easy. Some anger is righteous and deserved, while other hostile expressions are inappropriate and even destructive. From a Christian point of view, when you focus on God in your anger instead of on the circumstances, you are better equipped to direct your anger at the offense rather than at the offender. In this way, you can actually take steps to restore a relationship rather than condemn and tear down the individual.

Abraham Maslow theorized that depression can stem from the lack of self-actualization. This is our inborn tendency, he said, to make the most of our potential or our natural gifts. People become depressed according to Maslow, when they are abnormally frustrated in their attempts to live up to their potential.[5] As you can see, these views of depression tend to stem from emotional trauma or stress, often occurring earlier in life. Today, doctors still validate those factors, but they are taking their research much further.

More recent studies suggest a biological basis to many forms of depression. Even Freud, in his day, speculated on the chemical properties of depression. Evidence points to deficient levels of the neurotransmitters norepinephrine, serotonin or dopamine in depressed people's brains. (The media seem in recent years to have homed in on serotonin as the prime culprit, though it isn't the only one.) There is still a debate in the scientific community as to why some people's levels of these particular chemical messengers are low. Many doctors now believe this has been shown to be a genetic tendency, although that doesn't account for all cases. Mark Gold, M.D. in his book, *The Good News About Depression*, cites statistics which indicate that in families where there is one parent with a history of depression, the children have as much as a 26 percent greater chance of becoming depressed, themselves. Where both parents have experienced depression, the percentage increases to 46 percent.[6] But what causes this predisposition?

There has been a long-standing debate over the degree to which depression is attributable to either a genetic tendency or environmental factors, the so-called nature vs. nurture debate. It is fairly obvious that children reared in homes where speech and thought patterns are consistently negative will tend to emulate those patterns themselves. There is scientific research showing the association of repeated negative mental "programming" (in simple terms, the mind operates as a computer does) with neural pathways in the brain. New evidence also indicates that recurrent depression may be a neurodegenerative disorder that disrupts the structure and function of brain cells. *Psychology Today* reported extensively in April 1999 on some new neurobiological findings in depression research. There is apparent evidence that nerve cell connections are destroyed in depressed people's brains, but indications that they can also be rebuilt.[7] Is this purely genetic or do our own actions influence it? No one really knows. Antidepressants and electroconvulsive or shock therapy (ECT) may aid in stimulating the generation of new neurons, thereby opening new neurochemical pathways in certain regions of the brain. Whether depression is genetically or environmentally induced, there is ample evidence of biochemical or neurological disturbances in depressed people's brains. At issue is how best to control or reverse them.

Because damaged nerve circuits connect to many other areas in the brain, depression is a whole body experience, which is why it can defy diagnosis for some time. It seems as if every fiber of the depressed person's being is affected by a general malaise. It takes some kind of catalyst to set the whole process in motion, usually acting as a time-delayed fuse, either genetic or environmental or both. Doctors are agreeing today that childhood factors do play a role in the onset of depression.

Depressive disorders strike all across the age spectrum, with an increasing risk factor for the elderly. Senior citizens comprise 13 percent of the U.S. population, but account for 25 percent of all suicides.[8] Both suicide and homicide rates for adolescents and teens have risen dramatically in the last decade, as well. Across the age spectrum suicides are nearly 60 percent more prevalent than homicides, however, according to U.S. Public Health Service statistics that rank taking one's own life eighth on a national scale of leading causes of death. It is the third leading cause of death for those 15-24 years old. That doesn't include the more than half a million people who unsuccessfully attempt suicide each year.[9] There is an indisputable crisis today with teenagers — adolescent boys, in particular. Our nation has been shocked by the eruption of murder/suicides particularly on school campuses in recent years by seemingly nonviolent youths. The truth is these unhappy, antisocial youngsters were crying out for help, but their cries went unrecognized or unheeded until it was too late. Shooting sprees by depressed adults made headlines in 1999, also.

The Gothic movement, perhaps an outgrowth of the Punk movement, is one of the means through which disillusioned young people choose to express themselves. They dress in sinister, black garb and listen to dark, eerie music. People worry that these youths are potentially violent, either to themselves or others. A national news service profile described a 19-year-old "Goth" as having the word "APATHY" tattooed on her upper chest in Gothic letters. She spoke of her paranoid obsession with death: "Dead people can't hurt you." Still others, including those within the movement, claim they are no more harmful than the Beatniks or flower children ever were. Normal, harmless behavior? I suppose time will tell. Close friends of mine who rode out this angst period with their teenaged son would argue there is nothing harmless in these movements.

I must caution parents of depressed adolescents who are uncertain how to help these children. First, realize the danger in denying there is a real problem. Withdrawal, sadness and anger may not just be an adolescent passage or developmental phase. If there is a family history of depression, you may need to seek professional help. Don't just wait for it to pass. Though we now live in an age where social stigma should no longer prevent a family from seeking help, it often still does. Youngsters needn't fear being told to "snap out of it" or feel their only recourse is to turn to substance abuse or unhealthy friends to find temporary relief any more than adults should. If we as parents, teachers or church leaders don't help them, they will likely get the attention of social misfits or deviants posing as concerned mentors, or they will simply end their miserable existence. Public awareness of depressive disorders and other forms of mental illness is still not where it should be. One mother whose son's life ended in suicide said in a recent news story "I did not know depression was a disease that could be treated." Such stories have prompted the Surgeon General to announce the first full scientific study of mental illness and to undertake a large-scale public awareness campaign aimed at suicide intervention.[10]

One can't help but take note of a highly publicized case where concerned and loving parents brought their daughter back from the brink of utter despair which was leading her down a path of violence and self-destruction. Cassie Bernall, one of the students slain in the Columbine High School shootings in April 1999, had written letters to friends in which she fantasized about killing her parents and herself. Her parents, galvanized in their resolve through their Christian faith to love and save Cassie, took drastic measures to bring her back. Cut off from her former friends, Cassie was enrolled in a Christian school and made to attend church youth group gatherings. Highly resentful at first, she was radically changed through the influence of her new friends at a church camp. She became a shining example of hope and inspiration to others and is considered by many to be a martyr. When confronted by her teenaged killer in the school library at Columbine and asked if she believed in God, her affirmative response became her last words. Her unwavering commitment inspired a revival of faith across the country, especially among youth. Ironically, she had once been on the same dark path as her killer.

Depression is real and it can be debilitating at any age. It is sad to see professing Christians give inadequate or outright incorrect advice to friends dealing with depression, either their own or a family member's. Yes, there are spiritual origins of depression (we're all prone to it when we're alienated from God), but depression doesn't necessarily point to some unconfessed sin in our lives. Nor does it mean we are lacking in faith. That is far too simplistic a view.

Living with a depressed person requires some vigilance. In the case of elderly depressed people, you must ask point-blank if they are considering suicide. They rarely take their own lives on impulse, as younger people do. Just knowing you are that concerned can break down barriers of stoicism and lead them to help. Silence and withdrawal bear looking into.

Know that there have been, and probably still are, some oddball theories about what causes depression. There are those who maintain, despite an abundance of evidence to the contrary, that depression results from a learned process that certain people using it as a means of escaping reality or responsibility undergo, as I mentioned previously. Perhaps this came out of a misinterpretation of Carl Jung's explanation of the balance between the conscious and the unconscious. Jung, known as the refiner of modern psychology, said in an essay appearing in *Modern Man in Search of a Soul* (1933), "The psyche is a self-regulating system that maintains itself in equilibrium as the body does. Every process that goes too far immediately and inevitably calls forth a compensatory activity. ... The relation between conscious and unconscious is compensatory."[11]

It is still unclear to the medical community why some people who appear to be genetically predisposed to depression don't succumb to it while others who have no apparent genetic predisposition do. New ways of studying how the brain functions are already beginning to yield more answers to these and other questions. I strongly suspect one of the answers has to do with an individual's thought and speech patterns and the way he chooses to process (based on temperament or social conditioning, perhaps?) information internally. Dr. David Burns, a pioneer in the development of modern cognitive therapy, has said that "depression is not based on accurate perceptions of reality but is the product of mental slippage: Depression is not a precious, genuine, or important human experience. It is a phony, synthetic counterfeit."[12] Burns defines 10 common cognitive distortions in his book, *Feeling Good: The New Mood Therapy*, that are worth taking a look at. While I tend to agree with him, I maintain that depression can also be the means through which we come to realize our human limitations and our need to rely on God's divine counsel. In this sense, depression most certainly *is* an important human experience.

One of the newer frontiers in medicine is the study of the relationship of the emotions and the chemistry of the immune system. Candace Pert, Ph.D., a research professor at Georgetown University Medical School and former National Institutes of Health pharmacologist, said in an article appearing in *Prevention* Magazine in 1994, "Our research has shown that emotions are intimately connected with the entire physiology of the body. The chemical processes that mediate emotion occur not only within our brains, but also at many sites throughout the body — in fact, on the very surfaces of every single cell."[13] Dr. Pert's earlier studies led to the discovery of endorphins, the body's internal mood elevators. The eventual discovery of endorphins in the immune system sent shockwaves throughout the scientific community. Dr. Pert has done research on neuropeptides or chains of information-bearing amino acids that exist throughout the body. They work by attaching themselves to any willing receptor, thus forming a communication network. "These neuropeptides — at least 60 have been discovered so far — are extraordinary, because they trigger emotions,"[14] believes Dr. Pert, though others do not yet believe her research to be conclusive. Nevertheless, when you see how we humans are the sum of our sophisticated parts, you understand more clearly how various patterns can be programmed into our conscious and unconscious thoughts.

Choose whatever theory you wish. We have to conclude that depression is on the rise, despite modern advances in medicine. In March 1999, *U.S. News & World Report* reported on the state of depressed individuals in our society, pointing out that some researchers are calling this an "Age of Melancholy." Some statistics say depression — and not just awareness — has doubled since World War II. Researchers point to more stress, fewer family and community ties and even nutritional deficiencies. If current trends hold, depression will be the world's second most disabling disease by the year 2020. Heart disease is still number one. The World Health Organization (WHO) already ranks depression first among women. Yet it only receives about 10 percent of the federal funding that heart disease research receives. What is disconcerting is that as many as three out of 10 depression sufferers (there is some disagreement on the numbers) apparently are not helped by any of the antidepressants on the market. Their illness is referred to as "treatment-resistant depression."[15] It isn't clear whether these people have tried cognitive therapy or psychotherapy or are just looking for a quick fix.

When you consider the other social problems that are related to depression — drug and alcohol abuse or acts of violence, for example — more focus on depression's causes and treatments is clearly justified. To that end, President Clinton announced recently that he is seeking more funding and research for the treatment of mental illnesses. Tipper Gore has become a spokeswoman for this cause, admitting that she once underwent treatment for depression after her son was involved in a serious accident. Whether or not this Presidential emphasis on mental illness can slow the runaway train we call managed care and begin to turn it around remains to be seen. It could, in fact, speed it up. Yes, we need to increase public awareness and education, and many of our mental hospitals need to be overhauled. In many ways, the system has run amuck. "Funding and research" don't always provide the correct emphasis, however.

Part of the problem is that depression is not just one disease with one course of treatment that generally controls or cures it. Doctors often refer to the disease as "the depressions" because no two cases are exactly alike. Depression can seem as complex as each individual. Perhaps those who see themselves as created by an infinite God stand a better chance of finding relief from their unique illness. It is comforting to believe that someone, somewhere understands what makes each one of us tick. The term "healed" evokes a different reaction than the term "cured."

Though we are limited by our human qualities, I believe we are no less magnificent than the universe God created to sustain this imperfect human race. We are a microcosm of the cosmos, which is not limitless, as some people imagine it to be. Everything God created is finite. Only the Creator is infinite. Some scientists today maintain that the universe was constructed only for the purpose of sustaining life on planet Earth. That idea rankles those who are determined to find life in the cosmos. We still have discoveries to make about the microcosmic universe God put inside each of us and how we can utilize His marvelous creation within and without for the purpose of healing our minds and bodies.

Dr. Shad Helmstetter, noted author and lecturer, cites an interesting scientific observation in his book, *Network of Champions*. It seems that while neuroscientists were researching Alzheimer's disease, they accidentally uncovered the secret to reversing negative mental "programs," which, unchecked, can lead to depression and other mental illnesses. Helmstetter is well known for his mind-computer analogies. What was that secret? In a word, hope. "What the researchers discovered not only confirmed that our programs are physical pathways in the brain; they proved we could do something about it," says Helmstetter. "They learned that if a person could somehow stop using an old program long enough, the old program would actually break down chemically — all by itself! And the change is physical in the brain, measurable with sophisticated medical imaging computers."[16] In other words, new neural pathways can be forged in the brain through cognitive therapy, not just electrical or biochemical therapy. Now the relationship between psyche and soma becomes more clear, showing us the old axiom "we are what we think" isn't just self-help mumbo-jumbo. The mind-body connection has long been recognized in the scientific world. For a while, it was called the "placebo effect," referring to the improved health of people who are unknowingly given little more than a sugar pill in medical studies.

If we are what we think and we realize our thoughts can lead to undesired actions and sickness, how can we learn to think correctly? Dr. James McCullough, a psychologist and professor at Virginia Commonwealth University, whose 20 years of work in studying the chronically depressed had led to a therapy model claiming 85 percent success within three months of treatment, says he teaches patients to live in the here and now, with responsibility for their actions. "The people I work with have lived with depression for years and years, and it is unremitting," explains McCullough. "Time has literally stopped for these people." He shows then through his unique therapy, which is built around an interpersonal relationship between patient and counselor, the effects of the way they live. "People who for years have said it doesn't matter what they do begin encountering the consequences of their behavior," adds McCullough.[17] The antidepressant-only group of his study experienced only a 50 percent recovery rate, which should be news of interest to the many psychiatrists relying on managed care options for their patients. McCullough found a high success rate with combined drug and psychotherapy. He admits, however, that maintaining that recovery is his great concern.[18] I reiterate that the missing link lies in the spiritual realm and in the support system that family and/or friends, particularly those in the religious community, can provide.

Another psychiatrist and author whose viewpoint begs attention is Stephen J. Bergman, M.D., Ph.D. Writing under the pen name Samuel Shem, Bergman has written two novels based on his experiences in the field. *The House of God* was Bergman's revelation of medical training practices in a hospital. *Mount Misery*, published in 1997, takes the story into a prestigious mental hospital. "As in *The House of God*, the things you would think were the most fictional are the most true," Bergman told a newspaper reporter, adding "Study after study shows 80 percent of people who walk into a psychiatrist's office have no clear biological illness. ... I'm concerned about how many people are taking drugs for psychiatric problems when what they really need is someone to talk to."[19] Like

Dr. McCullough, Bergman is targeting managed care and the bottom-line-profit mentality of HMOs.

The human mind is intricately complex and there are parts of it we haven't begun to fully understand. When we observe something that appears to help people make changes that heal and make them whole, we can either accept that we are on to something or we can reject it. It's our choice. Sometimes we stumble onto truths that we didn't know existed yesterday. Such is life's journey. I don't believe that God intentionally wants to keep us in the dark about those things we haven't yet discovered. He is the author and creator of all, and as such, does not have to reveal His purpose for everything that happens. Science and faith carry us farther when they are interconnected. As you will see later, controlling our thought processes is no less than a biblical command. (Read Proverbs and the New Testament books of James and Philippians, for starters). When we change our hearts we change our minds and, ultimately, our health. Sometimes the mind leads in this orbital process that comes round and affects the heart and overall well-being.

The relationship between depression and other physical illnesses has been recognized for some time. In 1992, *Prevention Magazine* published an article called "10 Physical Reasons You May Be Depressed." Citing a number of researchers, the editors list the most common physical causes of depression as being:

1. Prescription drug side effects
2. Thyroid problems
3. Premenstrual Syndrome (PMS)
4. Other female hormonal disturbances
5. Diabetes
6. Rapid weight-loss diets
7. Lack of exercise
8. Sunlight deficiency
9. Inadequate nutrient intake
10. Inadequate carbohydrate consumption

The article goes on to say, "Nearly one-third of all people diagnosed with [depression] may be suffering from a physical illness masquerading as an emotional problem." In fact, there may be as many as 75 hidden physical causes of chronic depression.[20]

Now, the point must be made here that nearly everyone has experienced some degree of the symptoms I've listed earlier at some point in their lives. This might be termed "existential depression," which can be considered a normal response to life's frustrations. You can be depressed to some extent and still be functional. There are a host of situations we encounter at any given time that can cause us to be depressed, but as the circumstances change, the fog usually lifts and we feel "ourselves" once again. Excessive grief over the loss of a loved one or a relationship or other traumatic experiences can cause temporary depression. If this type of depression lasts too long, it may be necessary to seek counseling or even medication for a while.

Today when I find myself facing situations fraught with anxiety the worst that will happen is that I may lose a little sleep or get somewhat irritable, whereas before I was rendered nonfunctional and ultimately needed medication to make it through. Two times in my recent devotional reading I have been led to similar metaphors recommending prescriptions of faith for anxiety. The first was a story built around a pastor who felt his congregation were pumping him dry. An older, devout woman reminded him that in such times, he simply needed to sink the "pipe" deeper: "You need to get down where there is water again." The second metaphor came from planting and growing. A middle-aged couple decided to put their entire life savings into an apple orchard, despite the risks involved. Sure enough, their second crop was 90 percent destroyed by a late spring frost. Despondent at first, they remembered they had agreed to trust God for the harvest. The wife said, "Every morning, I had to sink my roots deep in my faith, where anxiety couldn't reach."[21] There are circumstances that can cause the strongest of us to lose our grip temporarily on faith. But when we discipline ourselves to keep on bearing up under the pressure, God promises to see us through our pain. However, no one realizes more than I the difficulty in programming discipline into a sick mind. It can be like trying to run a program on a computer that's infected with a virus. You know what it should do; you just can't make it happen sometimes. With many forms of depression, is just isn't possible. That's when you need help.

David Seamands, author of a book called *Healing for Damaged Emotions* says that depression might be God's method of "cruise control" for your life when you get unbalanced with life's activities or find yourself overloaded with stress.[22] I believe this could have been true in the case of the friend with whose story I opened this chapter. But I prefer to let her doctor or pastor make that judgment.

It generally takes an experienced doctor to determine whether or not an individual's symptoms point to clinical depression. If depressive episodes come and go without any clear cause and are severe enough to render a person nonfunctional (episodic), or if a person remains depressed for long periods of time (chronic), then he or she is most likely experiencing clinical depression or Major Depressive Disorder. Again, a qualified doctor's judgment can best determine that. Long-term treatment, usually psychotherapy and medication or — in the most extreme of cases where an individual is deemed a threat to himself or to others — hospitalization may be in order.

One of the more recent developments in the mental health field was the establishment in 1991 of an annual National Depression Screening Day (NDSD) by the National Institute of Mental Health. In 1996, approximately 100,000 people were screened at this event by some 18,000 health professionals across the country. The numbers increase every year. The goal of NDSD is to identify people suffering from clinical depression and refer them to treatment. About one percent of those screened usually are hospitalized immediately. This program has recently been expanded to include an anxiety disorder screening day. An April 1998 article in *People* Magazine stated that as many as 65 million people have anxiety-related problems. On average, about 70 percent of patients screened for depression from 1991 to 1996 needed some kind of treatment. Dr. Douglas G. Jacobs, the Harvard psychiatrist who founded the program, said in an article appearing in *Parade* in 1996, "I estimate we have saved about 7,000 lives."[23] In 1997, after more extensive analysis and perhaps because of increased awareness of the annual screenings, he more than doubled that estimate in another *Parade* follow-up story. Your local mental health association or a local media source can tell you when an upcoming screening day is scheduled.

According to a study concluded in 1994 — the National Comorbidity Survey (NCS) — psychiatric disorders, including depression, are more prevalent than previous studies indicated. The study reported that nearly 50 percent of the respondents (ages 15 to 54) experienced at least one lifetime disorder while close to 30 percent experienced at least one one-year disorder. More than 17 percent of the respondents had a history of Major Depressive Disorder and more than 10 percent had experienced an episode within the past year. The figures are higher, of course, when you take into account the elderly population. The NCS showed that, compared to men, women tended to have a higher rate of affective and anxiety disorders while men had a higher rate of substance abuse and antisocial personality disorders.[24]

The NCS researchers found that most people with psychiatric disorders did not receive professional treatment. Less than 40 percent of the people with a lifetime disorder had ever received treatment, and less than 20 percent of those with a recent disorder had been in treatment during the past year.[25] Such statistics are sad when one realizes that treatment for most psychiatric disorders is highly effective. People don't have to suffer. In fact, success rates of treatments for major mental disorders, and particularly depression, range from 60 to 80 percent while the most common treatments for cardiovascular disease have success rates of only 40 to 50 percent, according to former National Institute of Mental Health Director Frederick K. Goodwin, M.D.[26] These figures may contradict the public's general misconception.

Today, the most-employed treatments for major depression are either drug therapy, psychotherapy or ECT. There are other natural treatments, as well. In Germany, the herb St. John's-wort (hypericum) is prescribed for depression by doctors more than any synthetic drug, including Prozac, and now it's catching on in the U.S. Science has also uncovered another form of ECT. It's called "rapid transcranial magnetic stimulation" (RTMS). This method of brain stimulation is more accurate than ECT. The long-term effects are unknown, but this treatment may be available for general use in two or three years.[27]

The most common type of treatment in the U.S. for depression in recent years has been a combination of drug therapy and psychotherapy, such as I underwent. There is a trend in today's managed health care programs, however, toward referring patients to one form of treatment or the other for economic reasons. I still believe many people need both, at least initially. Most patients will respond to some kind of antidepressant, and there are new ones coming on the market all the time. Those who don't may find ECT or RTMS effective.

Scientists are working to develop tests that may determine which depressed patients will be unresponsive to medication based on certain types of brain activity. Three major types of antidepressant medication — cyclics or tricyclics, monoamine oxidase inhibitors (MAOIs) and lithium — have been successfully used to alleviate symptoms of depression for 35 years. All these, however, have varying degrees and types of side-effects. Two newer categories of antidepressants called selective serotonin re-uptake inhibitors (SSRIs) and serotonin and norepinephrine re-uptake inhibitors (SNRIs) are currently receiving wider distribution among depressed patients. Prozac, the first of these, was approved by the FDA in 1987 and still leads the way in prescribed drugs for depression and anxiety disorders, though many doctors feel it is overprescribed and in doses that are too large. And, it has not proven to be the magic pill it was touted to be. Its cousins are Zoloft and Paxil. There are still no long-term studies on Prozac's or any of the other newer drugs' effectiveness. Doctors often combine several different antidepressants or vary dosages throughout the day to achieve more effectiveness or counter side effects. A more pure form of Prozac is about to come on the market, and research is currently being done on a new antidepressant called MK-689 which targets "substance P," a compound found throughout the body that is believed to play a role in depression.[28] This new drug is reported to have fewer side effects than other antidepressants.

Some people may be fearful, as I was, of submitting to some type of antidepressant drug. I have long been a person who preferred natural remedies to synthetic ones. However, the success I experienced with the medication I used dispelled my fear of properly monitored drug therapy. Doctors are prepared to employ various types of antidepressants until the most effective one with the least side effects is found. Ultimately, it's your choice. Some people opt for depressive episodes over unpleasant side effects. Most feel that side effects such as a dry mouth, morning drowsiness, nausea or some sexual dysfuntion are far desirable in the short haul to the symptoms of depression.

Antidepressants are intended to restore normal mood levels and activities, including sex drive, although some, especially the newer SSRIs, curb sexual desire or cause sexual dysfunction. Some are appetite stimulants while others seem to lessen the appetite. The appetite suppressant effects of some antidepressants led to the diet pill mania we recently witnessed giving rise to the controversial drugs fenfluramine and phentermine (fen/phen). Prescribed like candy for a while, fenfluramine drugs bit the dust when the FDA pulled them off the market because of dangerous side effects late in the summer of 1997. Hopefully, the publicity surrounding these ill-fated drugs hasn't sullied the reputation of the legitimate ones that have helped many people to overcome or function with depression. Perhaps this adversity will cause more people to pursue "talking" therapy, which according to numerous studies has been shown to be as effective as, if not more effective than drug therapy. Cognitive therapy or therapy aimed at helping patients to change their way of thinking has a very good track record. It is related to what Norman Vincent Peale called "imaging." This finding coincides with Dr. Helmstetter's beliefs, as we saw earlier (remember the chemical basis of changed mental programs). The difference is, cognitive therapy can render permanent benefits, not dependent on the ongoing biochemical effects of a drug. An important word of caution: please tell your doctor if you are taking any herbal remedies to avoid the possibility of interactions should antidepressants be prescribed. Doctors should routinely ask if you are taking any other medications or herbs.

Depressed or anxious people who are not receiving treatment from a psychiatrist or psychologist are, in some cases, being prescribed minor tranquilizers by other medical doctors, because of misdiagnosis or the lower risk of side effects. Unfortunately, they also are running the risk of addiction, a far worse consequence. My mentally ill brother knows this danger firsthand. He and I are the only siblings in our family who have experienced major depressive episodes. Our temperaments are the most similar. My brother compounded his problem by abusing drugs and alcohol for many years. His clinical diagnosis is schizoaffective disorder, bipolar type, and he has not recovered in more than 25 years. While doctors recognize his illness as difficult to treat, if not altogether resistant, I'm afraid he hasn't helped his cause much. He has been uncooperative much of the time and has used his illness as an excuse. There is little doubt that much of his psychosis has been drug-induced — some of it possibly by prescription drugs. He feels he is a victim — and there may be some truth to this — of the recommended medical protocols in various hospitals which prescribed a plethora of drugs for him over the years. Was he merely a human lab rat? The body of knowledge about mental illness has increased dramatically over the years, but often, necessarily and unnecessarily, at the expense of patients. Still, it's hard to fault doctors for trying various courses of treatment. In most cases, they're doing the best they can. Drug research always gives patients and doctors new hope.

For a brief time at the age of 39, my brother began desiring to take charge of his life and question the need for the various medications, which had begun to include the highly addictive Librium. He counseled with physicians who had conflicting opinions. Changes were slow in coming. He finally gave up trying to fight. It was clear that he was making great strides forward when he chose to be proactive, but he may have overreached and eliminated medications that were helping him. Now it is heartbreaking to watch him simply wait for his life to end. His experience has left me frustrated with some standard medical practices. This is why I suggest that a person seeking treatment for depression carefully consider the doctor or doctors you will choose and do all you can (or enlist the help of a family member) to research your condition independently. There are legitimate doctors and counselors and there are merely "shrinks." Some doctors do not take into consideration the chemical effects of past recreational drug use in depressed patients. Yet, there are medical data to suggest that drug abuse, even after detoxification, permanently lowers a person's serotonin levels. It is believed that serotonin production can be restimulated by certain natural agents in cases such as these or by the therapies I mentioned that regenerate neural pathways in the brain. I contrast my brother Greg's experience with that of my father. My dad recently told me he was most in danger of having his spirit broken during his times of hospitalization. He holds the record at a Virginia state mental institution for the most escapes. He just couldn't stand being there. He submitted to various medications because he had little choice, but he knew his real problem was alcohol. Since doctors felt compelled to render a diagnosis, he was classified as everything from paranoid schizophrenic to manic-depressive. My dad's moment of truth came when he was prescribed lithium for what we today call bipolar disorder (manic-depression). He never accepted that diagnosis (prophetic of my later plight when a doctor gave me the same false diagnosis). He made a decision to stop taking the lithium, bringing himself off gradually. "I threw the rest of the bottle in the fireplace one day and watched them burn," he told me. "That was it for me." My dad never saw the inside of a mental hospital after that day, except to visit my brother. I don't relate his experiences to frighten anyone away from hospitalization. It is sometimes necessary. My dad threatened to commit suicide from time to time. Any hint of suicidal tendencies will land a depressed person in the hospital where close supervision is easier.

In order to give a balanced view of scientific evidence relating to treatments of depression, a word must be said here about vitamin or nutritional therapy. As early as 1947, Tom Spies, M.D. recorded his success with niacin supplements in patients suffering from depression and anxiety disorders. He concluded that insufficient intake of niacin could definitely be the cause of some forms of depression, and wrote his opinions in a book called *Rehabilitation Through Better Nutrition*.[29] In 1962, further credence was lent to this theory by Abram Hoffer, Ph.D., M.D., then president of the Huxley Institute for Biosocial Research in New York. In his book, *Niacin Therapy in Psychiatry*, Dr. Hoffer describes impressive results of studies conducted with large doses of nicotinic acid, a form of niacin, that he gave to depressed people.[30] I can add here that a great-aunt of mine died in a mental institution the horrible death of pellagra, long known to be a result of niacin deficiency. Its latter stage is insanity.

Doctors and nutritionists have not generally followed the niacin trail in more recent history, but they have gone on to follow up these pioneering studies with others, also discovering vitamin B-6 and the amino acid tryptophan, essential in the formation of serotonin, whose role in mood disorders has been fairly well-established, could benefit depressed patients. Another amino acid, tyrosine, has been shown to be effective in the treatment of depressed patients who had a deficiency of the neurotransmitter norepinephrine. Effective vitamin therapy for depression, according to some researchers, includes supplementing with Vitamins C, folate, biotin, bioflavonoids, calcium, potassium, magnesium and B complex. Some nutritionists caution against excessive amounts of vitamin D, zinc or copper. Caffeine, they say, should also be avoided or consumed in small quantities. Increased protein intake has long been said to be beneficial to depressed people. I used to reach for a banana when I was feeling low because I knew it was high in protein and potassium. Actually, bananas are reputed to contain beneficial levels of serotonin and norepinephrine and would appear to be one of nature's natural remedies for depression. Women, in particular, have long known there is a correlation between their moods and cravings for chocolate, the age-old comfort food. It turns out that has a scientific basis. In addition to the serotonin-enhancing sugar and fat, chocolate contains chemicals that affect neurotransmitters connected with mood. Siberian ginseng is also known to be a natural mood elevator and chamomile, long the leading herb prescribed by doctors in Europe, is known for its calming effect. Omega 3 oils, especially those from extreme cold-water fish, are also being shown as effective in treating depression.

Ongoing studies in nutritional and herbal therapy may prove to yield more conclusive results in the future. I have watched the recent fad phenomenon known as the high protein, low carbohydrate diet craze with interest. I, too, believe carbohydrates have been overemphasized in our recommended diets over the years, but more of a balance is needed than either the carbo or the protein gurus appear to advocate. It will be interesting to note whether any measurable differences in depression occur by those following this regimen. I think my mom was right: "Moderation in everything; nothing to excess." And husbands, it's okay to give that occasional box of chocolates to your wives. You'll both be happier for it.

Since I have become aware of exceptional cases of healing of all sorts of physical maladies by homeopathic physicians, I began researching the efficacy of homeopathic treatment for depression and other affective disorders. I have a strong, personal interest in alternative medicine, which I feel has been underrated. Also, I like medicine which doesn't merely treat symptoms, but considers the whole person, as homeopathy tends to do. It stands to reason that if a person can activate his body's natural healing response, he can marshal these forces against mental as well as physical illnesses. Homeopathy is a system that treats disease using minute quantities of substances that in massive doses cause the same symptoms being treated. Modern Western medicine is considered allopathy, which seeks to cause an opposite reaction to symptoms being treated. There are a number of reputable, skilled homeopathic doctors who have a good track record treating depression. The frustrating thing is that the traditional medical and psychiatric communities won't always cooperate with homeopaths in this type of healing effort. Large pharmaceutical companies are one barrier. It's simply not profitable to market non-regulated medicines, although there is a branch of the FDA that approves some of them. Antidepressants are big money makers for the large companies that develop them. I believe wholeheartedly, however, that this is the next medical "frontier" waiting to be explored and that somewhere down the road, there are answers waiting in this arena for many people suffering from all forms of depression. Even the NIMH has recently studied alternative medicines. Eventually, the medical community will have to give way to viable research and take note of the anecdotal evidence, if government and pharmaceutical lobbyists don't get in the way.

Nutritionist Michael T. Murray has written a number of books on alternative healing and natural remedies for depression and stress-related disorders. In *Stress, Anxiety and*

Insomnia, he details the efficacy of several natural healing agents, one of which is St. John's-wort. He also has high regard for Kava root extract and L.72 Anti-Anxiety, a homeopathic medicine.[31]

While I am grateful for the response I had to pharmacological treatment, I know, as statistics indicate, that not all people will respond to most antidepressants. Trazadone or Desyrel is really almost in an antidepressant class by itself, incidentally. Some may continue to feel strongly about subjecting themselves to drug therapy. Desyrel can cause priapism in men (persistent, abnormal penile erection), and there is a range of side effects that can and usually do occur in all patients to some degree. I was fortunate to have very diminished side effects. Perhaps that is because my lifestyle forced me to do many other things right.

I found I was going against the grain of traditional medical protocol when I requested to be taken off my antidepressant medication. More than that, historical evidence was against me. But there is a point at which traditional medicine and I tend to part company. Spurred on by my brother's anguish with medicine, I did it anyway and succeeded. Not everyone will have the response I did because belief systems and personal motivation will vary. My doctor can't say exactly why I walked away from treatment and have remained emotionally healthy for more than six years after a 15-year battle with Major Depressive Disorder, but I can. It was because I wanted it as much as I wanted the next breath of air. It's no great mystery. Why do cripples get up and walk even after doctors have told them they can't? I also happen to believe one or more intercessors are faithfully praying in the case of such healings. Prayer and an unconquerable will to recover are the recipe for what we call miracles.

Most doctors believe that severe depressives will require lifelong, intermittent treatment. Everyone's ultimate goal is healing, even though it may not be attainable in all cases. Some of us may have to settle for management, as with diabetes or other diseases. You can live with neurological or biochemical imbalances. In any case, you will be better off with your spiritual house in order. When your soul is at peace, you *are* healed. The most significant recovery from depression occurs in the emotional and spiritual realms. Perhaps God chose to heal me totally so that I could become a messenger. My recovery certainly had more to do with internal thought processes and prayer than with external, chemical agents, but the two often work in tandem.

Of course, there are other avenues of relief and healing available outside traditional or holistic medicine. There are several types of counselors with both Christian and secular backgrounds who are qualified to guide a depressed person through psychodynamic therapy aimed at resolving underlying emotional conflicts that most certainly contribute to their depression. I believe this type of therapy is very likely essential to recovering long-term mental health for many depressives, but — and this warning bears repeating — it also can be risky in the hands of the wrong "professional" care-giver. Also, it takes longer to recover with psychotherapy than it does with cognitive therapy, which uses a more direct approach. Many people just lack that kind of patience. In truth, some of the aversion to psychotherapy may be justified. It's a hard word to define. I believe some methods of psychotherapy are overrated, and some therapists actually exacerbate their patients' problems through the power of suggestion. Some counselors allow their patients to go on in frequent therapy sessions long after this intensive care should be necessary. Therapy should be self-limiting ultimately, otherwise it just becomes another addiction.

Good counseling still can be invaluable. Qualified counselors come from the fields of psychiatry, psychology and licensed clinical social work, for the most part. I consulted counselors from all three categories. Some counselors are also ordained ministers. The pastor of your church, if you attend one, is usually a good referral source for qualified counselors. Don't be afraid to check the credentials of the persons you are considering. Are they board-certified? Do they stand in good repute in the community and with their colleagues?

Some people may choose to join a support group of their peers that is led by a lay person, usually someone who has experienced depression and has overcome it. These people have an insight into the types of feelings you may have because they've been there, themselves. Remember, they are lay people, not doctors. Most of these are religious support groups. Often, those involved are led to examine the Scriptures for specific references that are helpful. Prayer is an important part of recovery in the support group setting. In the group I belonged to for a while, we were encouraged to journal so that we could get in touch with our feelings. Often, a depressed person only knows pain, but has difficulty in specifically describing what type of pain it is. The journaling exercise helped me to identify the pain factors in my life so that I could target my recovery toward those specific issues. Another important benefit of journaling is establishing a personal history and a record of how you've overcome. Being reminded of the successes you've had leads to anticipation of more success. This exercise reminds you that God is in control, even when you can't see the top of the mountain. Peer support groups offer an atmosphere of acceptance that can often help break down barriers of fear and guilt we might have erected. Some clinics sponsor intensive weekend counseling and treatment programs. Incidentally, virtually all counselors accept forms of major insurance and many offer services based on a sliding scale to coincide with your financial circumstances.

In the days of my illness, hospitalization was recommended more frequently than it is today. Now, outpatient treatment while remaining integrated with society and regular activities is more the norm. I did contemplate hospitalization and perhaps I could have benefited from some in-patient treatment, but I was left badly scarred by the childhood memories of visiting my father and later, my brother in mental institutions. Even though that is not necessarily the kind of environment I would have been subjected to, it was a barrier I could not overcome. I made the conscious decision to remain plugged into my normal environment. There were strong factors governing that decision, in my case. One was my family. I needed the love and support my husband provided to me on a daily basis. Another was my church family. My pastor and his wife were key support people. Other friends prayed unceasingly for my recovery. My church activities provided me with a sense of purpose and continuity. I sang in the choir, taught Sunday School classes and led women's Bible studies. Even though episodes of depression caused me to have to table these activities from time to time, they were a mainstay of my life.

Russ and I had some mentors who were coaching us in biblical principles of marital and financial success. They recommended that we read some very helpful books, such as Norman Vincent Peale's *The Power of Positive Thinking*, Dr. James Dobson's *What Wives Wish Their Husbands Knew About Women*, Robert Schuller's *Self-love* and, eventually, Shad Helmstetter's *The Self-Talk Solution*, which deals specifically with changing mental paradigms through monitoring what we say to ourselves. We jokingly called our self-improvement program brain surgery. The truth is, we both had a lot of incorrect thinking to overcome. Because we had the opportunity to listen to a wide spectrum of people share their life or faith stories with us, we were given the assurance that we, too, could overcome our circumstances and grow into better and more whole people. And we did. It takes getting out of the sterile, clinical environment to realize this kind of growth. As Robert Schuller is known for saying, "It takes guts to leave the ruts."

Remember the familiar truism, "The best defense is a good offense?" That's the approach I tried to take in dealing with my illness as long as I was in a position to mount an attack. That could mean everything from educating myself on how to survive depression, soliciting prayer when I felt an episode coming on, learning to reach out to others who could help me (this was particularly difficult for me for a long time), identifying the factors that were catalysts to episodes of depression and cultivating an attitude of thankfulness at all times (another "toughie").

I can distinctly remember during my early years of depression those moments when I forced myself to punch through the wall of despair and fight my way back to the light. I think I actively tried to use my anger as a weapon against my depression at times. It became more and more difficult to sustain the huge effort of will necessary to fight through the darkness as the years wore on, however. I found myself having to rely more on others and on God. But He gradually showed me that what I perceived as my weaknesses actually could become my strengths. When I started allowing others whom I could trust to reach over the wall and help me over, I was getting closer to victory. When I allowed myself to be totally broken, I began to find healing. I knew it had to begin somewhere in the depths of my soul. I thought of myself as a battleground for spiritual warfare. The powers of light and darkness appeared to be alternately vying for my life. Russ will confirm that at my worst, I looked like a woman possessed by a demon. I'm not here to debate demonology, but I know that when I forced myself to look into my own eyes, what I saw frightened me. The tormented orbs looking back at me did not appear human.

The more prolonged a period of severe depression is, the more difficult it becomes to extricate yourself from the pit of despair. Unless you can find a way to head off an episode, or change your program, so to speak, you're probably going to have to ride it out. I prefer that people seek treatment which can alleviate depressive symptoms, but I know there will be gaps in treatment or times when particular therapies become ineffective. When those times come, it's necessary to be armed with defensive weapons to sustain you through the battles. In my case, I exhibited certain warning signs of impending gloom that were usually obvious to my husband even before I was aware of them. If he commented on my emotional state while I still felt I was okay, I was likely to become angry and defensive, all the while knowing he was right. Likewise, there were certain signs that only I knew about because they were so private and internal. I usually became particularly emotional, crying sometimes, but mostly when I was alone. I would verbalize my love for Russ and the girls repeatedly and feel very needy. I actually succeeded a time or two in abating a full-blown depressive episode at this point. If I didn't, the next phase would be emotional detachment. When my children were very little and I entered this phase, I literally could not respond to them. I did everything automatically, as if I were a robot, if I could do it at all.

Many times, stressful situations would lead me to anxiety or panic attacks. This is not uncommon for depression sufferers. I began to feel as if I were living my life at a high rate of speed. My mind would race, my heart would pound and I would imagine all sorts of awful things. In this state of paranoia, I believed people were pointing accusing fingers at my inadequacies. If my anxiety level became so high that I was unable to sleep, even for one night, I knew I was inevitably sinking into a deep depression of God-knew-how-long a duration. Not everyone experiences anxiety attacks concurrently with depression. People who tend to sleep excessively are more depressed, or hypoactive, than anxious and hyperactive. These nights of sleeplessness were the loneliest and most painful times I have ever experienced. I can easily see why many people choose death over this pain. Irrational fears took over every conscious thought. From that point until I was released from that incarceration in my emotional hell, my only concern was survival, both for myself and for my children. One of my greatest fears was that I would become a dangerously negligent or abusive parent. Prayer was the most effective weapon at this point in my struggles. To this day, I still wonder what memories lie deep in my daughters' subconscious minds. I pray that I have diluted any negative memories with the love and nurturing I have tried to give in great abundance since then. I am consoled with the knowledge that God can heal painful memories for them just as He did for me.

The ordinary stresses of life can become overwhelming burdens for people who are predisposed to depression. Maxwell Maltz in his book, *Psycho-Cybernetics*, said that we could all deal with stress more proficiently if we realized a simple truth: "that our Creator made ample provisions for us to live successfully in this or any other age by providing us with a built-in creative mechanism." Maltz said we get in trouble when we ignore this mechanism and try to solve our problems with conscious thought or "forebrain thinking." He illustrated his point with a reference to Jesus' statement in the New Testament that a man cannot add one cubit to his stature by "taking thought."[32] It's interesting Maltz used the term "forebrain thinking" in his analysis. Today's research centers largely around the prefrontal cortex (PFC) of the brain, which is the seat of emotions. The left side of the PFC is associated with positive feelings while the right deals with negative ones. Depressed people appear unable to activate the left PFC, as if the circuitry is faulty.[33]

The Apostle Paul, echoing Jesus' sentiments in his epistle

to the Philippians told us to "be anxious for nothing."[34] In Proverbs we are counseled, "Trust in the LORD with all your heart and lean not on your own understanding."[35] Christians know this "creative mechanism" Maltz describes as the indwelling Holy Spirit.

William James, the father of American psychology, wrote about the futility of worry in his essay, "The Gospel of Relaxation," advising, "When once a decision is reached and execution is the order of the day, dismiss absolutely all responsibility and care about the outcome." This, as witnessed by the great number of tranquilizers and antidepressants dispensed today, to say nothing of illicit drug use, is far more easily said than done.

If you see elements of yourself or a loved one in the symptoms I have described, I urge you not to take this lightly, but to seek out a diagnosis and course of action aimed at restoring emotional health. It took my husband getting actively involved in my treatment before I realized my most significant progress. Often, depressed people are incapable of helping themselves get the proper care. A severely depressed person is stymied by the decision-making process. Logical thinking is almost non-existent in this state of mind. Take the initiative to help a loved one get the necessary help if you must.

It is important to maintain as normal a relationship with a depressed person as possible. Avoid being critical or angry, though your patience may be taxed to its limits. Acknowledge that the person is suffering. Express affection and respect for the depressed person. Believe me, kindness is appreciated by someone in this state of mind more than you can imagine.

One more word of caution: please do not think you can comfort your spouse with sexual intimacy when he or she is depressed. When you're depressed, every part of you is depressed, including your sex drive. Even when you're taking medication, sexual dysfunction may persist. Don't take offense to the rejection of your advances. Intimacy will return in its own time.

Four

I recounted my ways and you answered me; teach me your decrees.

Psalm 119:26

~~~~~~~~~~~

A Heart's Quest

One of the more helpful techniques I employed to deal with my depression was journaling about my feelings. Several counselors had impressed upon me the importance of keeping a journal. My "official" journal starts on my grandmother's birthday. There must be some deep, underlying significance in that. In a way, it is related to the date that I stopped taking antidepressant medication for good, which happened to be my grandfather's birthday. My journal began in the early fall, September 17. Perhaps this signifies that a journey through winter was still ahead. The journey ended, for all practical purposes, in the spring several years later on May 17. Is this coincidental? Having been drilled in critical analysis in all my studies of literature, I still find myself looking for symbolic meaning in events.

I was about six weeks from giving birth to our second daughter when I undertook journaling. I had been struggling with renewed depression for nearly a year following the two-year hiatus I had mysteriously experienced. It was clear that this nightmare was not going away on its own. I was willing to try anything. My support group was an important step in my recovery. I felt a sense of acceptance there. I felt particularly close to the leader, who had experienced depression similar to mine. On my first day of journaling, I wrote:

"The sharing was really open and spontaneous on everyone's part. I felt a bond growing among us. I was so glad to be there. I had felt good on other Thursdays, but never so good for everyone in the group who seemed to benefit in some way today. I was so aware of how special Russ is to me because of his love and support and steadfast faith. He called me shortly after I got home and I told him how much he meant to me. I feel a special closeness to him right now."

I went on to write about some little struggles I was having and about concerns over my pregnancy.

September 18
Russ may be offered a high-paying job in Los Angeles. Should he take it? We don't know, but we don't have a lot of time to decide. I talked to Pastor Rick today. It's ironic he had called to say he had been thinking about us yesterday when I had felt the same thing about him and had wanted to call him.

September 21
I feel moody tonight, and I don't really know why. I can't point to anything in particular that is causing it. I do feel a little uneasy about the baby's due date and whether or not I'll have any help when the baby comes. Also a cloud of some uncertainty about whether we'll move, and if so, when, is hanging over me. I'm sleeping well. I think I'm eating a little too much junk food. I feel a little guilty because I'm not walking enough.

September 23
I slept well last night. Got a few significant things accomplished today. Russ and I spent some more time tonight talking about our prospects for employment, etc. We seem to be in virtual 100 percent agreement on things. I was really impressed tonight with a deep sense of the fullness of my life. I've been concentrating this week on living the moments of my days fully. Russ and I both take so much pleasure in watching Jennifer grow. She's a delight — so much personality, so much curiosity about the world.

October 19
As the birth of our baby draws closer, I'm feeling some anxiety about being prepared — the baby's health — how Jennifer

will react to a sibling — how I will be able to cope with the increased responsibility, especially in view of the possibility of being separated from Russ at the same time. When I put all this into perspective, I realize that all these factors are enough to make even the strongest of people anxious. I don't want to fall into an old familiar trap of feeling inadequate because I believe I'm strong, just human. I think I have come to know myself and what governs my moods and attitudes much better than I used to. I must make my watchword: PERSPECTIVE. As long as I can still see the forest and not only the trees, I can make it. I lay awake for about an hour early this morning thinking about it, realizing that I was very susceptible at that time to letting anxiety rule. But it didn't, praise the Lord.

October 28
Still no word on whether Russ will be offered the new job. This is the greatest source of frustration for Russ and me. Our patience is wearing thin. We had a very productive weekend a few days ago and got a lot done toward readying the kids' bedrooms, etc. We always manage to get it done, somehow.

November 12
Linda instructed us in group today in how to take care of ourselves, reminding us that we can't take care of ourselves in and of ourselves, without the strength of God. We must prayerfully seek His direction. We must do the tangible things, but pray always. Also, she told us that when we journal, we are building alters to God. (Note: Our second daughter, Natalie, had been born on November 4).

December 6
I called Linda. Her advice:
1. Read and study the Word, especially scripture references on fear and perfection.
2. Talk about my feelings and my history until I won't fear it happening again.
3. Make a list of all the things I want to accomplish and another list of what I can reasonably accomplish for the holidays.

4. Take care of myself, i.e. no sugar, plenty protein, enough sleep. Spiritual needs first, then physical.
5. Call on someone to pray for me (I did).
6. Accept what I can achieve for Christmas. Praise God for it. No perfection.
7. Give a loving attitude to my husband and children. Leave a legacy more important than striving for perfection.
8. Come to group Thursday.

There is a gap of about six weeks between journal entries at this point. This represents one of the lowest times of my life. I had contacted my support group leader early in December when I felt things were getting out of hand. Unfortunately, I was already too far into depression to be able to put her advice to use. It was a miserable Christmas, as the one before it had been. I feared I would lose my children, along with my sanity.

I'm sure it was only the prayers of others that kept me together. I was so low at one point that I can remember thinking that my children would be better off dead and I didn't care what would become of me. It was the first time I could truly understand how my mother must have felt when she contemplated taking our lives and her own at her lowest point. Coming out of that episode of depression made me see that nothing was impossible.

January 21

I'm waiting to go into Linda's (for group session). I arrived 10 minutes early. I took both kids to a new child care facility. Jennifer seemed to take to it right away, but cried just before I left. I'm concerned about her development right now because of the withdrawal she experienced following Natalie's birth and my depression in December. I don't want to put her through too many new experiences too fast. I just want to make sure I restore her faith in me. I want her to know I'll be there for her. I feel good about my relationship with Russ now. We're adults and understand and can communicate. I need to know how to communicate with Jennifer. Linda reminded me in group today I needed to take care of my little girl — me.

February 18
　　Today was a special day as I finally made it back to group following nearly three weeks of illness with the girls. I also got to see my new counselor for the first time. I felt an instant compatibility with her. I really feel fortunate that after years of searching and seeing doctors who had no real interest in me except in taking my money, I have finally found the right person. Thursday will be my special day each week. I was compelled to go through some old letters over the last couple days. I reread some letters from my mom and from Russ during the ordeal we faced in the Marines and after. Reading them gave me a warm, wonderful feeling as I realized how supportive and loving my mom had been instead of, as I had imagined, judgmental. That is an enhancement to my relationship with her. Russ' letters are like beautiful poems — songs, almost. Hardly a day goes by when I don't thank God for my husband. He is truly a wonderful gift and my dearest friend.

February 23
　　I need to journal tonight out of a growing sense of frustration — nothing major, but seeds of potential. These are the external factors, as I see them.

>　　1. First week of Russ working in Los Angeles. I'm on my own.
>　　2. Kids' illness and my need to rearrange schedules and stick closer to home.
>　　3. Not eating as well as I should. Too much sugar, not enough fiber.
>　　4. Having my period. Felt a little lousy yesterday; better today.
>　　5. Russ' daughter, Jessica has arrived for her two-week visit, even though we'll see each other on weekends, only.
>　　6. Not exercising. Can't go on walks with Russ not here. Can't fit into some of my clothes like I could after first pregnancy.

　　I fell victim today to one of my pitfalls when I start feeling frustrated: buying something for the house. Since Russ and I have talked so much about the importance of budget, I feel like he'll be mad when he finds out.

February 25
Linda says concentrate on the feelings you have just before you lose control — cry, yell, lash out, etc. That's what you have to deal with.

February 29
It seems there's a lot I want to write today — a lot of emotions I've experienced over the past few days. The weekend with Jesse here was great, even though it wasn't what I'd expected. Russ' ankle injury forced us to stay home all weekend. Saturday, I didn't see much of him (hospital four hours, slept four hours). Sunday was better. I was aware of feelings of resentment toward him for doing that to himself. I had to attend to him and his needs, as well as to the kids and try to get to know Jesse, all at once. I must say, I feel I did a pretty good job. By Sunday night, I was tired, but feeling good about the weekend. Russ was feeling better and truly wanted to make up for putting me in the position of having to work harder. He was later leaving so he could spend extra time with us. I enjoyed having Jesse here. She's very sweet and was very good with the girls. She wanted to make a good impression, I know, and to help all she could. I felt like I'd known her for a long time. She reminded me a lot of myself at that age. She has a sweet, pristine shyness about her that makes me relate to "my little girl." I'm aware of my fatigue today, and of how edgy that makes me. I feel I have the upper hand, though, because I've been here so many times before. I'm learning to overcome that urge to lose control, even though I've had a few battles today with that angry, inner me. Satan will not win this one!

March 1
I'm getting to bed too late for the second night in a row. It was a tough day — hectic because of outside intrusions and complicated by fatigue. I tried to slow things down by taking time out with the kids now and then. It seems there were so

many "straws that broke the camel's back" today, and I had a few angry outbursts — at no one in particular, and at Jennifer and even at Russ behind his back. Can't even remember what they were all about. I've been vacillating between feelings of love and concern for friends and family and feelings of anger. I realize I need to take better care of myself. I've prayed a lot today and want to leave everything in God's hands. As I lie down to sleep, my thoughts will be on releasing my burdens and on all the good I can think of. I have much to be thankful for. I will dwell on this. I love the Lord.

P.S. Have just finished my Scripture reading and was reminded to give thanks in all things, including trials. C.S. Lewis said, "God whispers in our pleasures ... but shouts in our pain."

March 9

I'm in bed early tonight (thank the Lord!) after a slightly tiring day of running Jennifer to the doctor and errands. She had roseola. I have a mysterious rash, myself. Perhaps poison oak I picked up from Russ' clothes. Interesting day, starting with an angry outburst I allowed myself to have with Mrs. "G" at the doctor's office. We, happily, resolved the misunderstanding and ended up laughing and hugging each other. Funny. Anger like that used to scare me. It was neat to see how quickly I could turn it around. The past week has been too full of events and I have most times been too fatigued to journal about them.

As I look back over my journal entries, I see a transition occurring at about this time. While I was still to face many more struggles, I believe I was experiencing measurable growth through this period.

March 12

Thursday was a good day. After a week of no group or counseling, I was ready for both. Good group session at Linda's. I shared my joy at overcoming my trials of the previous week. The peace at times was overwhelming. I feel I've made a quantum leap to a new me. I keep thinking of myself as a sword forged and tempered in a fire. I've been hammered into something stronger. I can rely on God more now for strength when I'd otherwise have felt alone. My friendships are becoming stronger and more meaningful. This is a real victory for me. I feel I'm becoming that transparent person I longed to become several years ago. God is truly replacing my pain and loneliness with joy and friendships. My earlier fears are disappearing. I feel free from so much of the past that has held me prisoner for so many years. There's still more release to come. That's where I'm directing my efforts in counseling. I still have concern about events of my childhood I may not remember — things that may have affected me deeply without my knowledge, things I may have repressed. Sometimes I think maybe there is nothing. Maybe it's just a feeling. But why would I feel it? I want to know. I am praying that God can take my anger, when I need to express it, and use it constructively. I thought of my healing the other day in terms of a healing wound that is scabbed over. It takes time — layers of skin — to form a scar. It will always be there, but the pain will be gone. If one chooses to remove the scab before it is ready, the healing takes longer. This is self-sabotage. The less we do this, the quicker the healing and the smaller the scar.

March 16

I just finished my counseling assignment concerning types of abuse I may have experienced in childhood. It wasn't particularly hard to do, but did bring back some painful memories and feelings. I remembered how I felt for a long time I'd never be able to have a normal relationship with a man because I felt so much pain and rejection from my father. Until Russ came along, that was the way it was. He helped me change all that. I do have some good memories of my dad, but it seems I tried so much harder to reach out to him than he ever did to me. I want to continue healing my relationship with my dad. I feel I've come a long way in my growth.

April 21

Group was supposed to be very special today since it's the day before Linda's and my mutual birthday. Maybe it was, and I didn't know it. I dragged myself there, like I did to reserve duty (Marine Corps) yesterday. Linda knew I'd been struggling. I'd reached out to her and to others in the group during the past two weeks. She homed in on me and confronted me in front of the group. I know she was right about some things, but she was too direct about it in group, I thought. I need to just accept myself in some respects, and change myself in others. I do have many fears, but I don't want to dwell on them. I want to confront them and deal with them and overcome them. Linda says I need to saturate myself in the Word.

April 25
It seems there are three mes: the one who rests easily at night; the one is hyperactive and needs little rest and the one who is an insomniac and needs, but can't get sleep. I slept last night for about six hours for the first time in two weeks or better. I awoke ready to deal realistically with my bouts of depression, from an emotional and physical side. I want to intensify counseling and stop group at Linda's for awhile. I can't use day care at the base anymore for the children. Jennifer is okay, but Natalie is not getting the proper care there. I must find something else, maybe someone who can come to our home. I need to describe my depression to (my counselor) — the great fear (panic attacks), the awful fatigue, the anger and being prone to violence, wanting to control the kids, etc. I will be talking to my doctor about my physical and spiritual state and about the use of antidepressants. Perhaps I really do need to see Dr. Hubbard. I need to talk in counseling about my self-sabotage — my fear of overcoming or succeeding.

May 11
Things to bring up in sessions:
1. Fears, anxieties — of people, new situations, motherhood.
2. Failures or perceived failures:
   - lack of femininity
   - money management (rationing food, etc.)
3. Lack of sleep and resulting crises
4. Naïveté — Feeling like a child in a woman's body.

5. Ability to appear "together."
  6. Anger
  7. Isolation. Don't want people to know how dirty, "unhomey" my house is.
  8. Comparing myself to others.
  9. Starting and stopping. Overcoming inertia.
 10. Feeling of gradually compromising myself away.

May 17

I had a good cry last night and today, and got some emotional release from both. I have felt deep pain and loneliness. The loneliness is not from being rejected, but from being the rejecter. I want so badly to reach out and love and let myself be loved, but I keep throwing up roadblocks to my own recovery. Several years of different types of therapy have helped me identify some things, but I haven't been able to get at the real heart of the pain I keep wanting to hang onto. Why? I feel God has blessed Russ and me in a number of ways, but in my times of darkness, I can only see the negative side.

There's a very practical prescription for keeping out of the pits: Try to eat, sleep, exercise, pray and practice positive thinking. These have all worked for me in the past. For two years, I was depression-free, though I did experience mood swings. I just decided I was going to take care of myself at all costs — that my life was valuable. I sang in the church choir. I tried to develop friendships. This is an area of deep concern for me. I can't seem to let myself get close enough to people to form real relationships. Russ has been the exception, but I'm not even always honest with him about my feelings or opinions. He loves me so completely and unconditionally, and I don't feel I can love him back that way. Yet, when I really let myself, I can feel great love for him.

The other great concern I have is for my children. I thought God would have been nice to give me sons instead of daughters because I would have felt less insecure with boys. But I have two beautiful girls, instead. I want to be a good example to them of a woman. I am so insecure in my role as a wife and mother that I fear I can't teach them what they need to know. Jennifer has gone through a number of my deep depressions (five since she was born) and has regressed in development each time. However, she has come back strong and still ahead of most children her age each time I recover. I've sensed hostility in her lately, naturally because I've been hostile. Today, that all seemed to change, somewhat. I think the emotional release of crying helped a lot. I was able to control my temper and largely ignore Jennifer's bad behavior and reinforce her good behavior. She responded normally. Natalie started crawling tonight, which excited me. She doesn't appear to be suffering much. Russ comes home in 11 more days. I feel more confident that I can make it now. I start doubling my medication tonight. So far, side effects are minimal. In my weeping, incidentally, I was remembering pain I experienced from my mom — belittling, lack of trust, pushing me to excel.

November 23
(Thanksgiving Eve)
I haven't written in my journal in many months, and feel a real need to tonight. Today was an unusual day. It started off terribly. I had been in such a down cycle for the last 10 days that I feared something terrible was about to happen. Russ has been stressed out to the max. We have argued, but mostly have just avoided each other. I slept very fitfully last night and had strange dreams. Lately, I've been escaping in my depression, and even in my dreams. I knew things would get worse and worse if I continued, but I actually didn't care.

I somehow managed to get out the door in my uniform and made it into the office 15 minutes late for an unscheduled day of reserve duty. Some kind of mysterious change came over me around mid-afternoon. I decided we'd have a good Thanksgiving. I went out and got a turkey and a few trimmings we still needed. Russ and I had a talk, not an argument — a blunt talk that I initiated — about my compulsive spending sprees and other problems. We started working toward some solutions.

I can't completely account for my change in mood today. We had a wonderful evening with the girls. They were so cute, and the change in them was remarkable. There are still many challenges, but I see daylight. I have hope tonight.

November 24

Great Thanksgiving Day! I planned and prepared by myself a large meal. The dinner was great — even on time. We enjoyed the parade on TV. We let Jennifer stay up to watch "Mary Poppins." I relived some of my childhood through it. Russ and I are continuing to talk through things.

December 6

I'm determined to make this a good day. I'll get must-dos done first. Thoughts of frustrations and irritations flash through my mind. As I go through the house and see things not done or half-done, I feel anger at myself and at Russ. His ability to improvise and solve problems is tremendous, and I'm grateful for it. But I get irritated when I think of all the times he's started projects and left them unfinished. He is willing to do the things we consider necessary for our ease of everyday living if I can meet him halfway.

January 18

My health has me concerned. I feel there is more biologically affecting me than I know about. I nearly passed out yesterday. I need a complete physical. I feel a ray of hope today, but am still very overwhelmed and isolated. I am looking forward to February and March because Russ will have more time at home. We'll be able to get more done and spend more time with the girls. My spirits are much higher tonight than they were this morning. I've been trying to sort out my anxieties. Yesterday, I felt such panic and dread that I faced my mortality squarely. When I stumbled out of bed in a stupor, I fell and nearly lost consciousness. I feared I would die. I managed to pull myself out of it (or was it God?). It was a dreadful experience. I know my physical condition could be crucial. I've come close to losing a will to live. But somewhere inside me I saw a small ray of light — something to hang onto. I cried out to God. I tried to pray in a calm manner. I finally was given a kind of calm and the vision to sort things out. It's amazing how sudden and drastic the mood change is. This has happened before. I need to be frank with Dr. Hubbard about my physical condition and my concerns. I seem to go into a panic as it gets closer to the time I'm to see him. I get a vision of poor, little me, hardly able to collect my thoughts and talk coherently. I feel that he must think I'm a hopeless case. I fear Angel sometimes thinks the same. But tonight, I have some insight and hope. I also feel an urging to confide at least part of what I'm going through to several friends. I feel a need to talk to my older brother.

January 19

I had a remarkable day today. I feel God was giving me some direction. After feeling better last night, I still was confused about how to handle today. Tonight, everything seems so much clearer. I'm not on overload, but on the contrary, I'm excited and hopeful. I feel I have a mission. I was pulled by some power (wonder who?) out the door late to the girls' class at the YMCA. The girls and I all enjoyed it. We needed the stimulation. I nearly canceled my counseling session. Thank God I didn't! It was one of the best we've had. I also had a good, open honest talk with Bonnie (the girls' baby-sitter). She was understanding and reassuring. It made us both feel so much better. I have established a routine with the girls for the evenings (dinner through bedtime). After bath time and songs, we go downstairs and pick up toys, then read books together. Then I rock each one a little, saying positive affirmations. Prayer time follows in Natalie's room so we can do it together. Natalie can finish her bottle while I rock Jennifer. It's working well so far. I feel good!

January 24

I still am confused as to why my emotional highs and lows are happening so close together. I feel very hopeful tonight, despite another low time this week. Too much of the time, I'm hung up on past failures. My thoughts keep me trapped in a cycle of fear and failure. I must overcome this at all costs. I realize I may have a life-long struggle with depression, but I have to know how best to deal with it. I know Russ will be supportive, especially if I'm moving in the right direction. My devotional reading tonight was about Elijah and his struggle to flee from Jezebel after she threatened to have him killed.

Pastor Rick used this story as an illustration to me once of how God can minister to our needs. Elijah was depressed to the point of death, soon after a great victory. But angels cared for him. God helped him get his perspective back. Today I feel my perspective coming back. I feel "connected" again.

My official journal ends here. It encompassed a time period of about 16 months during some of the toughest days I faced. While I had read through it several times over the years, its significance became even clearer to me as I transcribed portions of it for this book. I could see patterns developing in my illness, gradually bringing me more into the light of understanding. It was a full 18 months later that I finally came out of the long nightmare with the help of a different medication. Even without the journal, I still would remember some of the painful moments my struggle with depression caused me. But I'm not sure I could so easily remember all the little victories. Each was a milestone in my recovery. How thankful I am that I never have to walk that road again. I don't know what lies ahead in my life, however. There may come a time when I'll need my journal to remind me how I overcame as I am facing some new, painful situation.

Five

Anger is a wind which blows out the lamp of the mind.
                                              Robert Ingersoll

~~~~~~~~~~~~

I'm Okay, You're Okay ... Aren't We?

Our feelings have a great deal of influence over how we live our lives and interact with the world around us. We often lead with our hearts instead of our heads. How many times every day do you use the expression, "I feel ... ?" We feel tired, hurt, angry, sad, happy, loved, rejected and on and on the list goes. To have these feelings is to be human. To let them totally rule us is to let the tail wag the dog. The negative emotions often outweigh the positive ones. We naturally tend to be "wired" that way because we're products of a fallen (sinful) world. Common sense would seem to dictate that one shouldn't make important decisions based on emotions alone, but in post-modern society, feelings often rule.

Need an excuse? Geneticists are offering some new insight into our brain chemistry, and some new, possible ammunition for the insanity defense of our actions. Is there a gene that explains our often reckless, compulsive or otherwise unacceptable behaviors — an addictive gene, an anger gene, an anti-social gene, a manic or depressive gene? Instead of taking responsibility for our actions and looking for the cause of our emotional responses, we can all just claim we have a "shadow" mental illness. ("Oh, I don't have all six genes required for such and such a disorder, just two of them.") And if we're all just a little crazy, then really no one's crazy because pigs don't know pigs stink.

Let's hope planet Earth never arrives at such nonsense. By carrying that analogy to the extreme, I don't at all imply that we are to take lightly the role genetics play in mental illness. God created us each as unique beings and, alas, imperfect ones. But I do believe He gave us the equipment to overcome our weaknesses. In fact, the biblical concept of weakness isn't anything like the world's view. Historically, God has often chosen the lowly and the oppressed to accomplish His goals. "God chose the weak things of the world to shame the strong"[1] Paul writes to the Corinthians. He also tells them, "Therefore I will boast all the more gladly about my weaknesses so that Christ's power may rest on me."[2]

The natural law of cause and effect binds us to the consequences of being human and interacting with other humans. Early in our development, we begin choosing to respond in our own unique ways to various stimuli in our environment. Sometimes, after we've reached an age of accountability, we learn that our feelings in a given situation can cause us to be burdened with guilt. On a bad day at home with screaming kids, a harried mother may find herself wishing to be magically transported through time and space to a deserted island of peace and quiet. As soon as she allows herself to fantasize about such a possibility, she immediately feels guilty for even having the thought. On really bad days she may go so far as to wish she had never become a parent.

One of my favorite illustrations attesting to this frustration is the humorous poem, "Funny, Funny Mother," appearing in the book *Fresh Elastic for Stretched-out Moms*. A mother energetically prepares for Christmas and anticipates all the fun things she will do with her family. Gradually, her expectation gives way to holiday rush exhaustion and her children's conflicting expectations and she ends up being ushered to bed under heavy sedation on Christmas morning: "See Mother smile. ... Funny, funny Mother."[3] Every parent can relate.

Hopefully, parents facing mounting frustrations will take care not to verbalize those thoughts to their children, lest they respond with their own guilt for causing Mommy or Daddy not to want them. I know all too well how that works because I was the product of such inadvertent guilt-mongering. This was the one area in which I had the most difficulty cultivating forgiveness for my mother. I knew life was hard for her, and in all honesty, we kids sometimes didn't help matters. Children can be very selfish. I see this tendency in my two daughters all the time. We are born that way. But my brothers and I were sometimes left to feel that we were particularly bad and that we might indeed drive Mom to the brink of insanity, as she used to declare we would do. Having enough cases of confirmed insanity already on our family tree, we were afraid of adding one more. I thought I should have been able to invoke the biblical warning to parents — "Do not exasperate your children"[4] — as my defense. It didn't work. Told that I was not a problem-solver by nature, I became a bulldoggedly determined young adult who believed I just might be a more worthy person if I could learn to solve at least a few of the world's problems. I had a tendency to play the part of a crusader. Perhaps that's why I became a Marine.

I clearly remember the day in my training at Marine OCS when I stood with a team of fellow officer candidates, contemplating the seemingly impossible Problem Solving Course. One scenario required us to use whatever field expedient means we could to transport a seriously "wounded" buddy across an array of obstacles. The challenge was heightened by the fact that we were not permitted to communicate verbally. I was appointed team leader for this problem. Suddenly I saw the words "not a problem-solver" flash in neon across my mind's screen. For a few moments, I froze in fear, finally broken out of my inertia by a gesturing classmate. Needless to say, we did a disastrous job on that problem. But that day, I made a decision. I would never answer to someone else's name. I would discover my unique God-given abilities and decide who I was.

While still at home, I had internalized the injustice of this and other accusations by steeling myself emotionally and looking forward to the day when I could leave. My brothers apparently felt similarly. My older brother — Mr. Responsibility — left home and married a minister's daughter just before his 20th birthday. That marriage is still alive and thriving today, I'm happy to say. It is built on a solid foundation of godly principles. My younger brother tried various living arrangements, but unfortunately turned to a life of drugs and unhealthy friends. He pays a dear price today for that "freedom." I seemed tied to home through my college years by my sense of responsibility (bred by guilt?) for helping Mom. That's what girls do, right? I have had to reclaim values I once misplaced. I felt quite motherly toward my "baby" brother, Jeff, when he was younger. He was just 12 when my mom left for her overseas assignment. Sadly, we've seen little of each other in the ensuing years because of the divergent paths of our lives. He became an Eagle Scout and graduated from a historic military school, but like me made choices that led to a failed marriage and an apparent rejecting of his Judeo-Christian values. Jeff is on the cusp of the Baby Boomer and X generations. He is married to his apparent soul-mate now and is the only one of us still living in another state. We drop hints for him to "come home" from time to time. I love all my brothers. We share a sacred history.

I'm not sure how my staying at home during college affected my mom's own sense of guilt. She felt for many years that the pain she endured in her marriage was God's way of punishing her for running away from responsibilities at home and marrying at the tender age of 16. Her parents were disappointed, but didn't appear to judge her harshly, at least outwardly. She didn't need for them to. She struggled with a self-imposed judgment, as Christians sometimes tend to do. My mom's emotional makeup was largely the result of the decision she made at a young age to control her feelings at all costs. She had grown up with a clinically depressed mother whose illness she resented for stealing part of her childhood. My mom simply had to grow up too fast. Who can blame her for wanting to leave home? I tried as a teenager and young adult to reason with her that her "sin" had not been nearly as great as she imagined, and that she had more than made up for her shortcomings with her godly life. Later on, in spite of myself, I found myself putting on that same cloak of guilt when I faced my own insurmountable problems. I tried rationalizing, but the pattern I had become all too familiar with since childhood was too well-ingrained. Like both my parents, I became an angry person. Often, I turned my anger inward.

As Bernie Siegel has observed about people, in general, "If

they can forgive themselves, they won't need sick minds and bodies. If they can't find enough self-love to grant themselves this forgiveness, then disease can be the atonement that finally releases them from guilt, after which they can finally allow themselves to get well."[5] There's little doubt that this assertion applied to me. Sometimes forgiveness of either a parent or yourself is truly needed. Sometimes it is perceived forgiveness for perceived injury or guilt. The many broken homes in America leave in their wake a plethora of unmet needs and both real and perceived guilt.

Are those of Judeo-Christian faith more prone to suffering from depression and other emotional ailments than those who practice other faiths — or no faith? God is no respecter of persons, and He allows all of us to endure pain. The difference is sometimes we of faith feel we are being punished for some sin in our life, and we wonder why we can't find healing when we are at least trying to do everything by "The Book." We rationalize that we should be able to find the solution to our problems, and when we don't, we heap more guilt on ourselves. It doesn't help when well-meaning friends point out these so-called truths to us, or implore us to have just a little more faith. Guilt has its place in our lives. Many times when we feel guilty, it's because we are. A guilty conscience can lead us to repentance, or it can destroy us. We all want to have clear consciences and peaceful souls. But some of us have become experts at inventing reasons to feel guilty. The world brings us enough suffering without us having to manufacture it.

Some of this unhealthy perception of ourselves had its roots in the turbulent passage from adolescence to adulthood. My children, who were still practically babies — or so it seemed to me — when I first began this book, are now standing on the precipice of that dark, lonely canyon of inferiority, as Dr. James Dobson refers to the almost universal pitfall on the road to adulthood. I fell into it at about age 12 and spent more than a decade trying to get out. Where did this tendency to feel inferior come from? It seems it didn't take long after the birth of civilization for social convention to set up a scale of exclusive criteria for success and acceptance. One of these is physical attractiveness. Another is intelligence. Yet another is lineage.[6]

In reality, Christianity itself can be held historically responsible for fostering an atmosphere in which people were prone to downgrade themselves, though none of this was ever implicit in any Christian tenet. One of the most misunderstood concepts in the Christian vernacular is that of humility. Robert Schuller in his book, *Self-love*, sheds some light on how this came to be:

> A great problem arose when an attempt was made to translate the Christian concept of self-regard into Latin (the first language in which the philosophy of Christianity was put into concrete form). A Latin scholar has said "There is no word in Latin which adequately expresses the sense of self-esteem which as Christians we ought to have." The Latin translators, reacting against Aristotle's concept of puffed-up pride, took the teachings of St. Paul and used the Latin word *humilitas* in trying to describe what we ought to think about ourselves. Unfortunately, the word *humilitas* was more descriptive of the idea of downgrading yourself, running yourself into the ground, saying "I am no good," with the inherent suggestion that if you ever think of yourself as a wonderful person and have a normal sense of self-love, you are being sinful.[7]

While ancient Rome gave the world many worthy concepts that have withstood the test of time, this is one legacy we could have done without. No wonder Latin became a dead language.

I have seen people, women in particular, who have fallen victim to this kind of thinking. People who grew up practicing strict, authoritarian forms of religion or Christianity are the most vulnerable to low self-esteem and excessive guilt. I have listened to many of them sob out their stories in support groups or Bible study groups. It is distressing to hear. And what is worse is that we Christians sometimes shoot our wounded! It was the Pharisees, the zealous, hypocritical, legalistic religious leaders whom Jesus classified as the greatest sinners of his day. Why? As Dr. Schuller says, "Under the guise of authoritarian religion, they destroyed man's sense of self-affection and self-worth."[8] There was no translation problem here. Rather it was more attributable to social or religious status and the tendency to exclude those who didn't measure up to their arbitrary, self-righteous standards.

Psychologists have long maintained that more than half the patients in mental hospitals would not need to be there if they could learn to resolve their guilt, whether genuine or bogus. They need some kind of godly dispensation, freeing them from self-flagellation. How sad to think that people suffer needlessly and even choose to end their lives because they believe so fervently in lies! Some are lies they tell themselves, others are lies that were told them by ignorant parents or other influential people. I lost a decade of wholeness because I believed the lies.

A basic Christian tenet is that Satan (yes, we believe this being is real) is a deceiver by nature. Jesus called him the "father of lies." In fact, his greatest deception is fooling otherwise intelligent people into believing he doesn't exist. The Prince of Darkness will use this and other lies to hold us in captivity until such a time as we allow the healing and atoning spirit of Jesus Christ to release us from our pain. When we offer the guilt of our sins to our Savior, He forgives us once and for all time. Through Him, we know the truth which makes us free. Our sins and past pains are cast into the depths of a vast, bottomless sea where, as the late Corrie ten Boom used to say, he places a "No Fishing Allowed" sign. Our forgiveness reminds us that we can likewise forgive others who have caused us pain. That little sermonette is what we call the plan of salvation. It's based on accepting, not necessarily understanding, the redeeming atonement of a perfect sacrificial lamb for an impossibly lost world hopelessly separated by choice from their Creator. Incorporating that belief into daily living has liberated more people than all the "protective" legislation and social programs of the world's combined governments ever will.

The great deception of depression is that it appears it will never end. As Rich DeVos wisely reminds us in his book *Compassionate Capitalism,* "After crucifixion comes resurrection. After death comes life. After hopelessness comes hope. ... the end of your depression may be just around the corner."[9] How many swimmers have attempted to cross the fog-enshrouded English Channel only to give up within a short distance of the opposite shore because they *couldn't see how near it was?*

Everywhere I turn I see more and more evidence of people wanting to have a spiritual belief system. Worldly systems are letting them down. Many are searching for spiritual roots that will take them on a journey in and out of various religions until they find the validity they seek. An ABC news special hosted by Peter Jennings in April 1998 cited the following statistics: 38 percent of people in America pray to God; 43 percent attend church or synagogue and nearly 70 percent are seeking a spiritual connection of some kind.[10] The math says that some people warming church pews and praying still feel disconnected, even though they're searching in the right place.

More than a century ago, German philosopher Friedrich Nietzsche made his infamous declaration that God was dead. Today, 2,000 years after the God-man Jesus walked this earth, an ever-growing number of its six billion inhabitants are finding meaning in submitting their lives to a savior they recognize as living. God is not merely alive; He is thriving. Some even say that our love affair with science is being supplanted by our fascination with things spiritual.

The flower children of the '60s who finally grew up (some never did) realize that peace and love are not the world's natural inclination. We are not inherently good, and change doesn't come from the outside. Depression is and always will be a natural consequence of a deep spiritual void. God created us to seek and know Him on the deepest of levels. Jesus said in his well-known Sermon on the Mount, "Ask and it will be given to you; seek and you will find; knock and the door will be opened to you."[11]

Too many of us for too long have been trying to open our own doors to peace and happiness. Actually, God never promised us a life of happiness. Peggy Noonan, former speech writer for Ronald Reagan and George Bush, pointed out in *Forbes* Magazine in 1992, "I think we have lost the old knowledge that happiness is overrated — that, in a way, life is overrated. We have lost, somehow, a sense of mystery — about us, our purpose, our meaning, our role. Our ancestors believed in two worlds, and understood this to be the solitary, poor, nasty, brutish, and short one. We are the first generation of man that actually expected to find happiness here on earth, and our search for it has caused such — unhappiness."[12]

A major shortcoming with secular psychiatry is that it deals only with *our* truth. Individual truth, which comes from environmental and experiential influences, is distorted by selective memory and perception. But when we apply God's truth in our lives, things begin to fall into place. Beth Moore, who writes and speaks about God's principles of freedom, says the weight of our truth alone can be enough to break us. Like so many others, she experienced an abusive childhood and repressed key memories that surfaced later in counseling. How do you know if a painful memory is bogus — merely a suggestion or a lie — or is real? According to Beth Moore, her memories fit into her life's equation like a missing piece to a puzzle, confirming everything she already knew to be true. If this isn't the case with you, you're not dealing with the truth.

Despite the readily available keys to unlocking our mental and spiritual dungeons, depression persists. There is no disputing the great impact that depressive illness has on our society. In *Compassionate Capitalism,* Rich DeVos cites research that shows "about 20 cents of every dollar spent by U.S. businesses on health care goes for mental health and chemical-dependency treatment."[13] I was part of the Employee Assistance Program for substance abusers and those suffering from mental health problems at the company where I last worked. DeVos goes on to cite, "One of the most cost-effective areas for preventive medicine programs, it seems, is mental health."[14] Depression and depression-related illnesses cost U.S. employers more than $20 billion annually, according to the National Institute of Mental Health. The irony is that job-related and financial stresses also can spawn depression. In today's expendable world, employers and jobs are frequently viewed, wrongly or rightly, as a necessary evil that must be endured for survival. Companies whose employers tend to be more compassionate, no doubt, see less anxious and depressed people within their ranks. Perhaps if someone conducted a bottom-line comparative study in this arena, employers would sit up and take notice. At any rate, they might do well to learn how to help restore employees suffering from anxiety and depression to health. Their companies' balance sheets just might look healthier, as well.

I'm afraid the money my employer spent on my recovery process went into that vast, black hole where many of our tax dollars seem to go. I benefited very little from the secular counseling I underwent through the Employee Assistance Program. Much more helpful for me were my later counseling sessions with Pastor Rick Savage. I'm convinced that a major reason for that success was the friendship connection, over and above his pastoral expertise. I knew that he and Vonnie cared deeply about me and my family. I didn't just revert to a faceless file when I walked out of his office. They continued to pray for me and we remained in relationship, week in and week out. As I've mentioned earlier, I see this type of support system as critical for full recovery.

Rick and I used to talk about feelings and the role they play in relationships, in particular. He helped me to see that feelings in and of themselves are neither good nor bad; they just are. David Seamands says of feelings, "They are consequences of a whole range of things that come out of your personality. No emotions are in themselves sinful. What you do with them will determine whether they lead you to righteousness or sinfulness. The emotions themselves are a very important part of your God-given personality equipment."[15] Feelings are automatic responses based on your own unique makeup. Once we learn that we can control the outcome of our feelings, we gain the self assurance that we are okay, no different from anyone else who experiences the same feelings. It is particularly important that, as parents, we teach this to our children.

As I stated in the opening paragraphs of this book, since birth, I have been equipped with intense emotions. People like me are probably more prone to depression. But like many children growing up in an ailing family, I tended to suppress my feelings associated with painful memories. Charles L. Whitfield. M.D., who wrote a book called *Healing the Child Within,* says that it is not unusual for children from seriously dysfunctional families to repress up to 75 percent of their painful memories as they grow to adulthood. He also says:

> Our feelings work in concert with our will and our intellect to help us live and grow. If we deny, distort, repress or suppress them, we only block the flow to their natural conclusion. Blocked feelings can cause distress and illness. By contrast, when we are aware or experience, share, accept and then let go of our feelings, we tend to be healthier and more able to experience the serenity or inner peace that is our natural condition.[16]

I'm sure I would have found great comfort in openly confiding my feelings and inner conflicts to a close friend years ago. But I really didn't have a friend like that, outside the various counseling relationships I was involved in. I got close to developing a deeper friendship with Vonnie, but I still saw her as my pastor's wife and I didn't want to become too intrusive. It's one thing to have a mentor or counselor and quite another to have a true friend or confidante. Today, I can see the value of this kind of friendship quite clearly since I have crossed that barrier and have formed close relationships with people whom I can trust. Vonnie is still one of them. I can understand the loneliness and pain of others who are handicapped in the area of forming close friendships. Wanting to reach out to others, but not knowing how is a terribly frustrating feeling. Now I place high value on friends because I know how they can keep us centered in the chaos of life. As Rich DeVos says, "The beginning of the end of that struggle is to admit that you are struggling, first to yourself and then little by little to people you can trust to walk with on the road to recovery."[17]

Psychologist Larry Crabb believes that his profession may be somewhat overrated, that the sciences of the mind may have become far too technical and hair-splitting. He devotes an appendix in his book, *Connecting,* to this discussion. He, too, places high value on talking out your feelings with a good friend, and says this may be as effective as seeking professional help for many people.[18] Sadly, alienation and the lack of close friendships is an epidemic in today's world, a fact that has worked to the benefit of the many counselors who have become our surrogate friends.

One day, I was leafing through an old college anthology of modern poetry and came across a poem written by Carl Sandburg which expresses much of the frustration I faced as I kept my thoughts and feelings to myself. It's called "Aprons of Silence:"

> Many things I might have said today.
> And I kept my mouth shut.
> So many times I was asked
> To come and say the same things
> Everybody was saying, no end
> To the yes-yes, yes-yes,
>   me-too, me-too.
>
> The aprons of silence covered me.
> A wire and hatch held my tongue.
> I spit nails into an abyss and listened.
> I shut off the gabble of Jones, Johnson, Smith,
> All whose names take pages in the city directory.
>
> I fixed up a padded cell and lugged it around.
> I locked myself in and nobody knew it.
> Only the keeper and the kept in the hoosegow
> Knew it — on the streets, in the post office,
> On the cars, into the railroad station
> Where the caller was calling, "All a-board,
> All a-board for ... Blaa-blaa ... Blaa-blaa,
> Blaa-blaa ... and all points northwest ... all board."
> Here I took along my own hoosegow
> And did business with my own thoughts.
> Do you see? It must be the aprons of silence.[19]

My life is so different today from where it was just a few short years ago, it's almost hard to believe I formerly could harbor the harmful, self-punitive thoughts that used to occupy so many of my waking hours. Yet, I did. I gradually came to see the harm in being alone with my self-destructive thinking and self-talk. My internal conversations were often like debates between my positive self and my negative self. James Allen reminds us in his classic little book, *As a Man Thinketh*, that "Men imagine that thought can be kept secret, but it cannot; it rapidly crystallizes into habit, and habit solidifies into circumstance." He goes on to say, "Hateful and condemnatory thoughts crystallize into habits of accusations and violence, which solidify into circumstances of injury and persecution."[20]

As I progressed in each phase of depression, my thoughts became more harmful. I hated all of my perceived weaknesses. I projected my hatred onto others, as well. My innocent, unsuspecting husband was often the brunt of my hatred. My attacks were subtle instead of head-on assaults because I could not bring myself to confront him on any of the issues I felt anger about. I kept it all inside, nearly exploding from the pressure of it all. I would have mock arguments in my mind, which may have helped to some degree by getting me at least to focus on my feelings. But it would have been much healthier for me had I been able to vent my anger out loud once in a while, within reason. I was afraid of how my husband would have responded. I didn't like confrontation because I grew up with too much of it. Russ carried his own private anger, as well. He did give voice to it from time to time as his frustration overwhelmed him, but his patience with me must have been heaven-sent. I watched him drop to his knees in prayer every night. I know he prayed for my recovery, but he also prayed for strength and patience. And God met my husband's needs while he was doing his best to meet mine. Sometimes, I just needed him to hold me and not say anything. I remember once crawling into his arms like a child when I was only able to say "I hurt" over and over. Russ was my husband, my father and sometimes the tangible embodiment of God all rolled into one.

I gradually learned through counseling where my anger came from, and how unresolved anger can lead to depression. I learned through reading some of the positive-thinking books I formerly pooh-poohed how to affirm all that was good in me. We concentrated only on those books that were biblically based. Russ and I each began to carry with us a little stack of index cards with affirmations or positive statements about each aspect of our lives, written in present tense, as if they already were true. I posted some of these on my bathroom mirror so that I would see them frequently. Naturally, I affirmed my physical and emotional health as well as my relationships with God, family and friends. I found this "reprogramming" or cognitive restructuring exercise extremely helpful. My thoughts gradually became less negative, less angry. No counselor ever taught me this, incidentally. I learned it through my reading self-improvement program and from the Bible, itself. This doesn't mean we belong to the "name it, claim it" school, a philosophy which is not biblical. You can call this affirmation therapy. It works.

Even today, I still carry the remnants of anger with me. But if I feel myself wanting to respond angrily to a situation, I try to give myself an opportunity to think it through. When I fail and lash out at my children or husband, I strive to apologize quickly. This is one thing my parents rarely could manage to do. I'm sure it would have been so much easier for me to forgive if only they had said "I'm sorry" when they blew it.

I believe that anger is actually a derivative of fear. Psychologists say that the only fears we are born with are the fear of falling and the fear of loud noises. All other fears or phobias are acquired through our experiences as we grow up and learn about the world around us — or the world inside us. We impose limitations upon ourselves as we consider our perceived shortcomings. Every generation alive today has its own brand of collective fear to deal with. Many Baby Boomers narrowly survived the fallout of the '60s "tune in, turn on, drop out" philosophy — the "me" generation. Boomers' parents and grandparents remember the Great Depression. The younger X and Bridger generations suffer the alienation spawned by the absence of their fast-track, career-oriented parents.

While some fears are real and undeserved, fear can also be a selfish emotion. Excessive fear is self-centered. The opposite of fear is not courage, but faith and love because they break down the natural fear barrier and cause us to focus outward, which leads to confidence and selflessness. Fear is not our godly inheritance, but comes from our old nemesis, Satan.

Perhaps you're familiar with the acronym for fear: False Evidence Appearing Real. We are told in the New Testament that "God did not give us a spirit of timidity but a spirit of power, of love and of self-discipline."[21] The King James version of the Bible translates the word for discipline "sound mind," which is a closer approximation to the Greek meaning. A sound mind means that you will have disciplined thought patterns or thoughts that can override fearfulness. Discipline doesn't come overnight. It takes practice. That's what cognitive therapy — reprogramming — is all about. We have the basic God-given equipment. We just need to learn how to use it. We may have to try many times and fail before we master a skill, such as riding a bicycle. The same can be said of mastering our own emotions. My husband can tell you, as can any veteran of war, that there is no one without fear on the battlefield. The hero is just as afraid as the coward, but he is disciplined not to run. If he falls, he'd rather fall forward. Armor wasn't made for the backside.

Norman Vincent Peale said there are two primary forces in this world: fear and faith. "Fear can move you to destructiveness or sickness or failure. ... But faith is a greater force. Faith can drive itself into your consciousness and set you free from fear forever."[22] Many times we live in fear of the unknown. We don't know what is just up ahead in life and we're afraid we won't be able to cope with whatever it is. If we can all just stop and realize that life is destined to be full of surprises (some of them good) and frustrations that none of us can control, we'll gain some sanity.

When I'm writing, I sometimes take a break and play solitaire for a few minutes. It can help me clear my mind and get back on track when I'm getting too absorbed with a topic or idea. One day I realized that life is remarkably like the game of solitaire. We have little control over how the cards are shuffled or how they are dealt. They fall; we play them. Life happens; we respond to it. Most of the time, the odds for winning solitaire are pretty even. You can play six games and generally win about half of them. Sometimes you'll get on a winning streak for no apparent reason. But occasionally, it will go the other way and it seems you just can't win a game. This is frustrating.

I generally won't quit until I've won because I have a competitive spirit. Sometimes we attack life, forgetting that the deck that day may be stacked against us. We forget that sometimes that's the way it has to be. Frustrations can come from all sides — from our children, our spouses, our jobs, traffic — from anywhere. If we didn't win today, we'll get another chance tomorrow. And so it goes. We don't run away and hide. We don't throw down the cards and say, "That's it! I'm never playing again."

Today, Russ and I have cultivated some new habits and acquired some new skills in our marriage, one of which is a healthier way of communicating than the one we were formerly accustomed to. We still have more to learn about each other's sensitivities, but our marriage is much stronger because we've come to know each other better, and we've learned to strengthen our faith. If there's an area we're still growing in, it's in realizing how past hurts that came from our relationships with our parents and others can still affect our own relationship. My husband has had to struggle most with overcoming a critical, somewhat cynical spirit and a perfectionistic nature which have contributed to some conflicts in our marriage. I must honestly confess I have some of the same struggles. If we didn't truly love each other, ESPN would be broadcasting ringside from our house! These confrontations often have taken me back to my childhood struggles with my mother, in particular. Facing her perfectionistic criticism was a source of pain for me when I was growing up. It formerly didn't take much for me to revert back to the childish feelings of humiliation and inadequacy that I remember all too well. Even though I am less vocal in expressing my cynicism, my thoughts can bleed out in my body language (a typically feminine trait) which is equally harmful to any relationship. I know, however, that all this is being healed. The past two years, in particular, have been a true watershed for us. It's sad to see husbands and wives give up on their marriages before this type of healing can take place.

All the crises Russ and I have faced together have bonded us in a stronger commitment to each other. When we realized that our challenges were attacks from the enemy in spiritual warfare, we learned to stand together, heart to heart, in defense against the onslaught. Earlier in our marriage, we were tempted to point fingers of blame at each other as if we were "the enemy." It was difficult for Russ to know in those days how to fight my illness without wanting to fight me. His best weapon was love. In the end, all the powers of darkness could not prevail against the simple acts of love he showed me on a daily basis. Those installments of kindness and devotion accrued to a sizable account from which I still draw today when I feel under any kind of spiritual attack. I never could have made it through the recovery process without my husband. One thing I have observed in people who come from rather large families with backgrounds of poverty and early hardships (such as Russ faced) is their large capacity for loyalty and love. Caring for each other was a necessity for Russ and his siblings. How thankful I am that this is the man I finally married.

Bernie Siegel relates in *Peace, Love and Healing* that Physician and philosopher, Hans Zinsser, reflected on how his own illness affected his view of life:

> My mind is more alive and vivid than ever before. My sensitivities are keener; ... I seem for the first time to see the world in clear perspective. I love people more deeply and comprehensively. ... I seem to myself to have entered a period of stronger feelings and saner understanding.[23]

That statement comes close to describing how I feel today.

Bernie Siegel has noted that the medical profession considers recovery from any disease to be a return to the predisease condition. In his patients who recovered from life-threatening diseases, he has observed "in fact, a transformation into something new. In my experience, the disease often opens one to a spiritual reality previously unrealized."[24] My own experience with depression validates Siegel's view. I had hoped to return to my "normal" self and regain that former level of mental health. Not only did I find that part of me again, but I went far beyond that to realize a new and deeper perspective of life in a spiritual sense. Such a transformation defies explanation. I believe that is because it is not limited to this physical world. Perhaps people who have near-death experiences know this transformation that can only emanate from the spiritual realm. Mythologists recognize these rebirths as journeys to the underworld and back, the metaphorical descent into the Jungian unconscious or inner self where one confronts his dark side and gains a deeper knowledge of self, a deeper spirituality.

Most religions or faiths contain some kind of rebirth myth, but only Christianity can claim an actual resurrection. Christ's descent into hell and subsequent defeat of Satan gives all believers the hope of new life. Many people have struggled for centuries to believe that. Either you accept it or you don't. The experience of healing is a metaphorical resurrection. It is literally impossible after experiencing a dramatic physical or spiritual healing to know life in the same way as before. In this sense, I feel blessed indeed to have gone through my ordeal, for God has revealed to me through it what I otherwise might never have known.

I may walk with a limp today, but I am healed. Based on my interpretation of Scripture, I don't believe it could ever be God's will for anyone to remain depressed because depression weakens or even kills the spirit, and the spirit is what ultimately connects us to our Creator. I believe He permits this affliction, sometimes to get our attention and to deepen our faith, but He gives us the weapons with which to fight it. On the other hand, healing of a physical ailment may not be in our best interest from a spiritual perspective (remember the Apostle Paul's thorn?). We can be crippled, dismembered or otherwise infirm and still live a godly life, offering hope and inspiration to others with or without infirmities as we live it. It's far better to be physically challenged than spiritually bankrupt. Those who place their trust in Jesus Christ realize that He knew human suffering. On the cross, He experienced excruciating pain, suffering and abandonment. It was superhuman suffering because he literally *became* sin, something we will never be called upon to do. As He prayed prior to His arrest in the Garden of Gethsemane, knowing what was to come, he was depressed "... to the point of death."[25] Yet, we share the hope of resurrection through Him.

I did not knowingly choose depression, but I have heard it said that depression may choose us. It may indeed be a gift, when properly understood. I did make choices in my life that may well have contributed to it — choices that may bear consequences for some time to come. I can't change my history, but I can change my outlook. And I can refuse to fish the waters that are off limits. So can anyone. If depression has to be the door through which you may enter a redeemed life, then be thankful you have a door.

Scottish author and preacher George Matheson, who was blind, said it best in this simple, but eloquent prayer: "I have thanked Thee a thousand times for my roses, but never for my 'thorn.'... Teach me the glory of my cross; teach me the value of my 'thorn.' Show me that I have climbed to Thee by the path of pain. Show me that my tears have made my rainbow."[26]

Six

Where there is great love, there are always miracles.

Willa Cather

~~~~~~~~~~~~

"Amor Vincit Omnia"

People change in an atmosphere of love, as Pastor Rick Savage used to be fond of saying. That statement, along with two Scripture verses, became almost a mantra — if you'll forgive my use of the term — for me while I focused on recovery. I could also look to the Latin phrase inscribed in my wedding ring which translates into "Love conquers all." It reminded me that Russ and I already had overcome much and that, side by side, we would overcome this, too. I also saw and felt love in action in the good Christian friends who lifted me up and prayed for me for so long. I had been so fearful of being judged by others when they learned of all the garbage I carried inside my head. My fears had kept me from allowing myself to get truly close to others, the partial exceptions being Pastor Savage and Vonnie. How could anyone love me? I even believed that Russ' devotion to me was strictly out of a sense of loyalty and decorum, and that even he really longed to be somewhere else. When he would tell me that he loved me, the apparent disbelief in my expression would cause a pain so deep to well up inside him that I could see it in his eyes. There are two kinds of suffering when a person experiences severe depression: the suffering in the individual with the illness and the suffering in those who love that person. Both types of pain are great.

Christ commanded his followers to "love the LORD your God with all your heart ..." and "love your neighbor as yourself."[1] In fact, these are the greatest of all the commandments. Surely the healing power of love is apparent throughout Jesus' ministry. A key phrase in Christ's commandment is "as yourself." We know we are to love others, but what about ourselves? What does it mean to love yourself? Perhaps many people think, as I did, that this is vanity. Far from it. Self-love is revering and protecting the creation of God with which you are most intimately acquainted — yourself. We are created in His image. If you love yourself, then it follows that you will love others. Likewise, if you are incapable of loving yourself, you cannot love others, which means you cannot fulfill the whole commandment and truly love God. Perhaps you feel, as I once did, that God erred in creating you with all your flaws. I had to ask myself at one point in my life just how much of my anger was actually directed at God. Incredibly, I was blaming Him for some of my problems! It wasn't until later that I realized the very weaknesses I considered flaws could actually become my strengths if I allowed God to work in my life.

What we may perceive in the cloudiness of depression as God's mistake is actually The Great Deceiver's masking of our self-worth, fooling us into believing we are not children of God, but instead some kind of cosmic accident. Low self-esteem, as we saw in the previous chapter, is one of our greatest pitfalls. Pop psychologists, overreacting to this legitimate problem, have spun off a new "me" culture, which isn't really helping matters. It sounds like the '60s reinvented. Now we have a lot of self-centered people who still don't esteem themselves highly, which is probably why kids are blowing kids away. Those who believe in the fallibility of human nature or free will (which was first played out in what Christians refer to as "original sin" or the "fall") also believe Satan knows our weaknesses and uses them to undermine our effectiveness. His greatest aim is to get us to stop believing in ourselves and in Christ's power in our lives or subtly to get us to succumb to that base side of our nature which we have difficulty acknowledging.

Carl Jung once observed, "What I do unto the least of my brethren, that I do unto Christ. But what if I should discover that the least amongst them all, the poorest of all the beggars, the most impudent of all the offenders, the very enemy himself —

that these are within me, and that I, myself stand in need of the alms of my own kindness — that I myself am the enemy who must be loved — what then? As a rule, the Christian's attitude is then reversed; there is no longer any question of love or long-suffering; we say to the brother within us 'Raca,' and condemn and rage against ourselves. ... Had it been God himself who drew near to us in this despicable form, we should have denied him a thousand times before a single cock had crowed."[2]

It is with this line of unconscious reasoning that many a person finds himself sinking into the mire of depression, unaware that he has fallen victim to the oldest scam of all time, at the hands of the most ancient of the ancient con artists. I find it interesting that some of the national opinion polls I have read report that many people claiming to believe in God and the existence of heaven on the other hand do not believe either Satan or hell to be real. The prevalence of disillusionment is all the proof needed of Satan's existence. While he is the embodiment of evil and rebellion, there is no great, cosmic struggle between darkness and light. Satan's ultimate defeat was foretold 20 centuries ago, his fate having been sealed with Christ's death and resurrection. He is temporarily spreading strife and unbelief among God's people. Heaven is the glory we inherit when we become followers of Jesus Christ. Hell is...well, use your imagination. Ultimate separation from God is almost too awful to contemplate, at least for those of us who can accept moral absolutes.

The prevailing worldview for many people today is still being influenced by Enlightenment thinking. Any rational man can reach truth through his own intellect, or by studying the collective intellect of others, according to this philosophy. Heaven can exist on earth. I think it's time for another Reformation. Syndicated columnist Cal Thomas was on track in his 1994 book, *The Things That Matter Most:*

> The "absolute truth" is this: By acknowledging the objective existence of God and sin, one recognizes something that is essential to the achievement of true self-esteem. That is because without a higher state — or better condition — to aspire to beyond

this poor, wretched, rotting one that leads to death, all notions of worth become temporary, relative, and ultimately meaningless.[3]

Philosophy has even entered the realm of therapy. Plato and Socrates are now "enlightening" the disillusioned. What will be next in this trendy age is anybody's guess. This trend is anything but new, however. Paul addressed the body of believers in the early church who embraced Gnosticism and the elevating of spiritual enlightenment above simple faith in his letter to the Colossians: "See to it that no one takes you captive through hollow and deceptive philosophy, which depends on human tradition and the basic principles of this world rather than on Christ."[4]

How do we reach people today with the "Good News" of redemption when many of them don't believe in eternal consequences for their behavior? I believe it is with the simple truth of the ages, not with trendy half-truths and syrupy, new-age (or old-age) rhetoric. Truth never changes. If this makes the message too narrow to appeal to the mainstreamers of today, I can't apologize for that. It's not the message that has to change; it's the hearts of those who hear it.

Much is made today of the need to find the appropriate means to communicate the doctrine of truth to the youngest generation — the Bridgers, as they are called because they straddle two centuries. It is reasoned that this youth culture does not have the ability to grasp ideas in the same way as their parents or grandparents did. I have two of these youngsters living under my roof, and I say they *can* hear the message of truth and moreover can act on it enthusiastically. It just isn't being spoken consistently and with conviction by enough parents. As Cal Thomas has said, this message needs to be "drummed" into their heads. It will not merely be "caught." Times have changed, yes. People generally haven't. Cicero's lament, *"O tempora, O mores!"* (Oh, the times! Oh, the manners!) could just as easily have been uttered today. Even a cursory read of the Bible will show us that people still find themselves in the same situations of old, having the same basic needs. Neither God nor His message to His children has changed. Some still get it, some still don't. No matter how creative we get, we can never invent truth. Still, I suppose that doesn't stop some from trying.

Is there any wonder so many people succumb to unnecessary fears and lies masquerading as truth, considering all the media messages that bombard us daily? Judeo-Christian values in recent years have been openly mocked and biblical truths vilified by the power and pleasure brokers who occupy center stage in our culture. To some, it appears we are growing a generation with largely no moral absolutes. I sincerely pray not. Yet all around us tolerance is the order of the day. Where tolerance used to mean giving people freedom to be wrong, today it more often means everyone is right. The truth is watered down. "What is truth?" we ask. "Does it matter?" Research by George Barna and Associates in 1994-95 revealed that 71 percent of Americans reject the concept of absolute truth. Even more shocking is that 62 percent of those claiming to be born-again Christians have also concluded that "there is no such thing as absolute truth."[5] We can thank the cultural elites (the "brain-on-a stick" variety, as one of my former pastors calls them), many of whom took over our colleges and universities a generation ago, for that legacy.

Sooner or later, what many believe is truth leaves them empty. Disillusionment and a lack of values have led to an alarming depression and suicide rate among teens. They have few worthy heroes to emulate. People who are well-grounded with deep, personal convictions based on the positive values of their youth are far less likely to get distracted and discouraged in life. Those values are instilled first and foremost by loving parents. In many ways, we have let down this generation. Polls show they are more anxiety-ridden and fearful, both of the dissolving of their families and for their safety in the world, than previous generations.

The more I read the news, the more indignant I become at those spineless cultural elitists of our day who are allowing our moral underpinnings in America to erode, including the family, long the basic nurturer of self-esteem. The founding fathers would wretch if they were here today to witness some of the perversions of their bedrock expressions of faith. While it is sad to see people unable to recognize their depression, what is worse is society's denial that we (particularly my generation, the Baby Boomers) have created a climate that has allowed this wound to fester among us in growing proportions. How? Most notably by attempting to replace God with the deity of Self. Our national moral deficit has created an emotional and spiritual vacuum in which, for many, life has no meaning or direction. Hence, despair on a wide scale, even among a good portion of those who try to adhere to traditional standards.

I believe, among other detours we Americans have taken, that the aging feminist movement has had much to do with the rise of depression in our society, certainly among women, if not even among men. Its original proponents were self-proclaimed victims of broken families, voicing their hurt and lashing out with political barriers to try to keep this hurt out of women's lives. This misplaced movement did more harm than good. Feminism may have at least partly leveled the playing field for men and women in terms of civil rights, but it can't make men out of women or vice versa. God forgive us for even trying.

Some years ago, Dr. James Dobson devised a study to determine the leading causes of depression in women, who outrank men in their struggle with this emotional crippler by two to one. By far, the women surveyed in this study indicated that low self-esteem was the greatest source of their depression. Dr. Dobson says in his book, *What Wives Wish Their Husbands Knew About Women*, that low self-esteem "has reached epidemic proportions among females, particularly, at this time in our history." Why? Because "their traditional responsibilities have become matters of disrespect and ridicule."[6]

Although the decade of the '90s has seen a slight shift in sentiment toward the stay-at-home mom, women still face great stress today with the responsibilities of home and career and single parenthood as real as ever. Women who call in to prominent radio talk-show gurus — at least those of more conservative ilk — often ask for advice on how to juggle career and family. Today they are being steered with increasing frequency toward staying at home with their children. It stands to reason that this dilemma causes women to face more struggles with depression. Rearing tomorrow's adults and leaders is more challenging and worthy of praise than any other career.

Yes, full-time homemaking has inherent pitfalls. It's all too easy for husbands and children to take wives and mothers for granted, heaping undue burdens on them. Mothers of young children can isolate themselves too much. A little appreciation and time off go a long way in the home.

Most women, if given the choice, want to stay at home and raise their children. One of the strongest, altruistic motivations for the spread of home-based businesses and other work-at-home opportunities is the desire to see wives and mothers come home from the work force to raise their children and still have the ability to earn income, if necessary. It's no secret that government is not the family's best friend. Earning power has decreased while taxes have increased. Two incomes are often required to make ends meet. More time is required on the job as cutbacks force workers to take on added responsibility. No matter how healthy the national economy may appear, financial and work-related woes account for much of today's marital conflict and resulting depression.

The divorce rate in this country, on average, has fluctuated between 40 and 50 percent in recent years. Yet among those spouses who unite in the common goal of building legitimate home-based businesses, the divorce rate drops to a scant one to five percent. That in itself is a significant statement about the vast challenges facing the two-career family. I applaud all entities that, like Focus on the Family, the conservative Christian organization headed by Dr. Dobson, are bending over backward to help families in all of life's situations to cope with marital and parenting challenges. The embattled family can use all of that kind of support it can get. I am for anything that will bring families together under an umbrella of integrity and shelter them against the pressures of life which can all too easily lead to pain-numbing escapes of one sort or another.

I am not forgetting men in this discussion. I recently spent two hours visiting with an old friend and school mate who had been hospitalized for depression following his divorce. As an attorney, he has seen the reality of custody battles in divorce settlements. Even though his was amicable as divorces go, the pain of being separated from his home and his young daughter was more than he could handle. Despite statistics, some experts say that women are really no more prone to depression than men, who face many stresses, themselves. Instead, they say, women are more apt to admit feelings of depression or seek professional assistance while men may be socially conditioned to deny such feelings or to bury them in alcohol. (My friend denies he's depressed. He says he's just "bummed"). Men are five times as likely to commit suicide as women, who talk about it more than they go through with it.[7] Men tend to stoically keep to themselves and have fewer close friends. Responsibility can weigh heavy on their shoulders. Most women know how fragile the male ego is. Women are child-bearers and natural nurturers who seem to feel needed more than men do.

Other researchers say that hormonal differences between men and women are the reason women are more prone to depression than men. Male hormones may actually make men more immune in general to mood disorders than women. Research on the possible antidepressant affects of gonadal steroids, particularly testosterone, is now underway.[8] Of course, women have long understood that female hormones account for mood swings that at times can be quite severe. Premenstrual, pregnancy and menopausal imbalances of certain hormones, particularly estrogen and progesterone, can definitely lead to depression in women. Nonetheless, though women suffer more frequently from depressive disorders, men are by no means immune to depression or to the demons of low self-esteem. Lack of self-love and psychosocial conflict are no respecters of the sexes.

There are few medicines more effective than genuine love from another person at restoring emotional stability to the depressed person. In this instance, a hug or a word of encouragement can literally save a life. We all need to feel connected to others, to know that we will not be abandoned. Like the towering, ancient sequoias in California that spread their root systems out in all directions to support each other, we are stronger when we have others to lean on, and when we allow them to lean on us.

Bruno Bettelheim survived two Nazi death camps. He observed later in life about some of his fellow prisoners, "If there was no or only little indication that someone, or the world at large, was deeply concerned about the fate of the prisoner, his ability to give positive meaning to signs from the outside world eventually vanished and he felt forsaken, usually with disastrous consequences for his will and with it his ability to survive."[9] Focusing even beyond human contact on divine love can raise our hopes and help us to realize who we really are: wonderful creations of God who are "just a little lower than the angels."[10] Most survivors of the holocaust had little more than their faith to hold onto.

The power of love crosses the ages, and many a poet has penned an ode to this the most enduring and bittersweet of emotions. Have you ever read the biblical Song of Solomon? Not long before the King James translation of the Bible was authorized, Shakespeare was a prolific writer on the topic of love. One of his sonnets particularly illuminates the power of love (I interpret it as both human and divine) over despair:

> When, in disgrace with Fortune and men's eyes,
> I all alone beweep my outcast state,
> And trouble deaf heaven with my bootless cries,
> And look upon myself and curse my fate,
> Wishing me like to one more rich in hope,
> Featur'd like him, like him with friends possess'd,
> Desiring this man's art, and that man's scope,
> With what I most enjoy contented least;
> Yet in these thoughts myself almost despising,
> Haply I think on thee, — and then my state,
> Like to the lark at break of day arising
> From sullen earth, sings hymns at heaven's gate;
>   For thy sweet love remember'd such wealth brings,
>   That then I scorn to change my state with kings.
>   Sonnet 29

I mentioned that two verses from the Bible were key in helping me focus on recovery. One was written by the Apostle John, the other by Paul during times of tribulation in his ministry of expanding the early church. "Greater is He that is in me than he that is in the world"[11] wrote John. "I can do all things through Christ who strengthens me,"[12] Paul wrote. This latter verse in its proper context means I can handle all things that come my way, whether successes or failures. There were times when I recited these verses over and over to shield myself against the enemy. Researchers such as Herbert Benson, M.D., author of *The Relaxation Response* and director of Harvard's Mind/Body Medical Institute, have noted that people who practice this kind of "meditation," particularly if it is related to their spiritual faith, achieve the greatest sense of peace.[13] Today, mainstream research from respected institutions is confirming what people of faith have known all along: that prayer can and does have a positive impact on the speed with which people recover from illness. Make no mistake. Over and above the tranquilizing effect of belief in a universal power, there is a supernatural force at work when we pray. Prayer is our means of acknowledging that we are not alone in the universe, that we are connected to our source, our Creator. God is unquestionably in control.

I took great comfort in knowing that a man of God as great as Paul could suffer from afflictions the same as I could. I often wondered what Paul's "thorn in the flesh" could have been. I began to think of my battle with depression as my "thorn" — something that had to be endured, but which drew me closer to God rather than alienate me from Him. If His grace was sufficient for this great saint, could it not also be sufficient for me?

I related to John in many ways. He was the disciple, along with his brother James, whose epithet was "Son of Thunder." I knew what it was like to be angry much of the time. Yet, he writes so passionately about love in the Bible that he came to be known later in his ministry as the "Apostle of Love."

On more than one occasion, I turned to my pastor for strength and consoling when the pain of my depression became too great to bear. Pastor Savage was well-equipped to handle my self-rejection and feelings of deep loneliness. I remember several times calling him on the phone and sobbing out my pain for what seemed like endless moments. I believe God placed him in my life because he had the ability to really empathize with me, having experienced some low times in his own life. Silly as it sounds, he used to have me literally put my arms around myself and imagine God hugging me. He had to get graphic with me because my illness could leave me feeling like a little child. He encouraged me to love myself over and over. He was the first person in the role of counselor to actually point out the major stresses in my life and the potential for breaking down. He helped me separate fact from fiction. When I saw the real facts, everything made much more sense. Under Pastor Savage's mentorship, I gradually began to get back to the truth and the values of my childhood. Before my descent into depression, while I was still in my early twenties, I recall having the very strong conviction that I had a purpose — a destiny — to fulfill. I had been fortunate enough to have had some strong, Christian influences in my life. Had those not been there, the road to recovery would have been tougher.

Bernie Siegel speaks more than once about the individual's destiny or "path." Disease, he says,

> is an experience and a metaphor, with a message that must be listened to. Often the message will speak to us of our path and how we have strayed from it, so that our life is no longer a true expression of the inner self, or ... we are no longer singing our own song.

Siegel says that disease often becomes the factor that motivates us to find our dream.[14] He quotes Arnold Mindell as saying, "A terrifying symptom is usually your greatest dream trying to come true."[15]

One of my dreams certainly was to heal my relationship with my parents. I received a great deal of insight from a book called *The Blessing*, written by counselors Gary Smalley and John Trent. The authors give some painful accounts of children who grew up in homes where parents refused to or were unable to affirm or "bless" them, with devastating results in their later adult lives. In most cases, the parents were incapable of understanding the significance of the blessing because they hadn't received it from their own parents.[16] It is through forgiveness and remembering the biblical principle of honoring our father and mother, no matter what the circumstances of our childhood, that many people — myself included — have been able to release much pain and suffering.

It wasn't until relatively late in my struggle to recover that my parents even knew anything of my trials. I wish I could have felt comfortable in opening up to my mom, in particular, but I was already well on the way to recovery before I was able to do that. One of the obvious obstacles to dialoguing with my parents was the geographic distance that separated us. My mom was halfway around the world most of the time. I was in California and she was teaching American high school students in Germany. My dad was at the opposite end of the continent in Virginia. I put so much pressure on myself to open up to them on the rare occasions when I saw them that I froze in fear instead. I was able to get a few things off my chest in letters to Mom, but she never knew the real extent of my problems during the times when I needed her most.

Because I have such a different outlook on life today, it is sad for me to contemplate the difficulty I had in sharing my pain with my mom. I do know that I was reluctant because of all the heartache she faced with my brother. She was preoccupied much of the time, and I didn't have the heart to burden her any further. I had a great sense of responsibility for my mom's well-being. I know now that those feelings were somewhat misplaced, but I could not overcome that obstacle years ago. That child-to-parent protectiveness is a family-unique trait (a guilt-borne dysfunction, really) that seems to have been passed on from one generation to the next in my family. My mother's generation always seemed to be protecting my grandmother. We found out she didn't need as much protecting as we thought she did. Naturally, I learned the same about my own mother.

I decided that since I couldn't go back in time and actually be "re-parented" — though I could, in effect, travel back in my memory and find good things to dwell on — I would do the next best thing: focus on parenting my own children in a way that I would have wanted my parents to raise me. I felt that giving of myself in this way would also have a healing effect on me. In Russ, I had the advantage of an added element to the parenting equation — a loving, nurturing father. I knew my daughters would have that essential love that I had not.

I think it's important to insert a note here for parents. As obvious and as simple as it sounds, loving your children unconditionally may not always come naturally. Parental love compels us to set proper boundaries for our children at an early age and to teach particular consequences for attitudes and behavior. (Read Proverbs for some sound advice). I believe self-esteem is in direct proportion to the value system with which one is reared. It can be difficult for parents who grew up in a home where both praise and admonition were meted out inconsistently to understand where to draw the line with their own children. If you felt you could never measure up in your parents' eyes or you were mistreated, you may tend to overcompensate in your child-rearing methods, or you may simply repeat old patterns. If you start early on the right foot and remain as consistent as humanly possible, you can instill security and self-assurance in your children. If you have to learn this later, then by all means do so. Even in cases where genetic predisposition is a factor, the overriding condition for emotional health in children that they will carry into adulthood is a secure relationship with their parents — and their observance of a loving relationship between their parents.

While you cannot credit or blame yourself for your child's temperament, don't take lightly the extent to which you can shape your child's emotional well-being. Even if your children are older, it's never too late to heal a broken relationship. I've seen incredible miracles in relationships that many would have given up on. A blessing from a parent's deathbed can even do wonders. A consoling thought to parents who have failed in some ways (and that's all of us, to an extent) is that many children grow up strong and amazingly centered, despite coming from some pretty shaky backgrounds. That doesn't let us off the hook, however.

During times when I was a normal, loving parent, I took great pains to make sizable deposits in my children's "love bank." I was determined to prove the childhood statements my mother had made to me about my having no mothering instincts were lies. I basked in the unconditional love my daughters returned to me. From the moment our eyes first locked in loving recognition following birth, there has been no feeling to replace the way my daughters have filled the child-shaped vacuum in my heart. I can't imagine anything that could ever change the depth of my love for my daughters.

I learned through the pain of trial and error that forcing myself to reconnect with those little lovers was a powerful way of bringing myself back to the real world I would depart from every time I sank into the pit of despair. When our children came into our lives, my illness took on a new dimension. Jennifer and Natalie were at once my greatest fear and my greatest blessing. The responsibilities of parenthood can be overwhelming, even to an emotionally healthy parent. I constantly fought off the demons of fear — fear that I would cripple my children emotionally or harm them physically. Russ used to say to me with great fatherly satisfaction that we were going to have the girls with us for a long time. Whenever he would say that, I would almost cringe. My battles with depression had caused me to foresee a long struggle where he saw a wonderful journey. Abdicating my parental responsibilities to Russ many times was traumatic for me as well as for my children. But I had no choice at times. When depression took over, I was incapable of connecting with humanity. I was without emotion, my behavior sometimes bordering on the catatonic.

The clearest and most painful illustration of the impact my behavior could have on Jennifer and Natalie is an incident that occurred when Jennifer was about 22 months old. She was verbally gifted, and talked clearly at an early age. I had placed both the girls in Jennifer's crib for their own protection during a particularly difficult time. I had retreated to my bed in a state of emotional detachment. I have never forgotten the words I clearly heard Jennifer speak to her seven-month-old sister: "We've got to get out of here, Natalie." Of course, they could no more leave than I could force myself to simply "snap out of it." I didn't want to create a prison for my daughters, and yet that was what I was doing. My chains of despair were engulfing my precious children who were helpless to break free. At least I had some choices, and I thank God that I was finally able to discern enough to begin choosing a different path.

I know God empowered Russ with the strength to take over my duties with the children. I know also why I was led to marry a man with unusual nurturing qualities. There are days when I feel overwhelmed with love for my family. Everywhere I turn I seem to see reminders of the powerful force that binds us together. A birthday or anniversary card from Russ, a picture Natalie has drawn for me with her unique inscription of love, a certificate Jennifer once invented for her sister declaring her a member of the "Sister Honor Roll" so she wouldn't be envious of Jennifer's accomplishments.

This very day as I sit here writing these words is one of those days. I always knew I was blessed in a special way by my family, even in the worst of times. It is impossible to overestimate the restorative power of loving family members or friends to someone who is suffering from severe depression. Moreover, it is impossible to even fathom the healing power that flows from a loving God to one who is lost in the cavernous darkness of despair. God promised those of us who love Him that His Holy Spirit would never depart from us. I am proof positive of the truth in that assertion. Though at times I couldn't even see the mountain, much less gain a foothold on it, I held onto a tiny bit of hope that His love would someday get me over it. More than once in my suffering, I felt God's loving touch; I heard His voice.

I clearly remember one night as if it were yesterday. I was on my knees, alone in our bedroom, crying pitifully to God that I no longer wanted to live. I was reviewing my life, wondering what had been worthwhile about it. I felt I was a burden to those around me and that my life counted for nothing. Then God clearly spoke to me, by presenting to me the image of one person in whose life I had intervened. Had it not been for me, that individual would have been a lost soul, came His clear communication. I didn't realize I had made that much of a difference. God clearly showed me that I had important, unfinished business — things that only I could do.

One reason I could dwell on the hope of healing so much was the knowledge that others were praying for me. I still find it overwhelming that people who, in some cases, were mere acquaintances would take time out of their lives and put aside their own problems to pray repeatedly for me. Some of these people were acknowledged prayer warriors. Most were just ordinary people who cared. The sum total of all those prayers, whether they came from family members or total strangers, was a safety net for me against a fall into the everlasting pit of darkness. There were times when I could *feel* the power of those prayers. I knew it was real.

I have read much about the power of healing prayer as performed by such well-known therapists as Agnes Sanford, Ruth Carter Stapleton, Francis MacNutt and Leanne Payne. The closest I ever came to experiencing that kind of healing prayer was during some of the counseling sessions I went through with Rick Savage. He is not a trained prayer healer, but he introduced that concept to me. We spoke of time as a continuum and of the power of Jesus Christ to go back to my childhood and heal the pain I had suffered. We went through some exercises of healing visualization together that were helpful to me and got me on the right path.

I never cease to be amazed at the remarkable healings of the inner spirit, as well as physical healings, that I read about in the writings of the people such as those I cited above. There are too many similar anecdotes for them not to be accepted at face value. I often wonder if my healing would have come much faster if I could have experienced this type of healing prayer therapy. Francis MacNutt, in his book, *The Prayer That Heals,* says that this healing prayer relies on two basic facts:

> 1. that Jesus was a human being like you, and that his humanity suffered in that very area where you need healing so that you might be healed.
>
> 2. that Jesus can walk back into the past and change its effects upon your present life in a way that neither you nor any psychiatrist can.[17]

Ideally, the kind of sharing at the deep level required for emotional healing should come in our closest relationships, like that between husband and wife, for instance. It doesn't often happen, however. As MacNutt says:

> Because it is so painful to share these memories and because it takes time to even try, many married people have never shared themselves at this deepest level. As a result, they don't really understand each

other. When one of those raw nerves that were exposed in early childhood is touched, the explosion of pain and anger that results cannot be understood without understanding the source.

He goes on to say that present relationships could be vastly improved if husbands and wives would take the time to share their past hurts and pray together.[18] It took some time for Russ and me to begin sharing in this way. Probably, our most significant sharing came after my healing from depression took place. During this time, we encountered many conflicts because I was feeling my way back to where we should have been years before. We had never really enjoyed a marriage of any great length that wasn't marred by my depression. Russ and I are both headstrong people, and consequently, it is easy for us to hurt each other by our words or actions.

We gradually came to see the benefit in praying together. We had prayed separately for years, Russ being far more faithful in prayer than I. There were times when we even prayed long distance over the telephone when Russ was away and I was struggling. Several close friends also prayed over the telephone with me when we couldn't be together. It is one thing to pray for someone, but another altogether to pray with them, and be able to use the healing power of touch along with the prayer. The power of the laying on of hands is demonstrated many times in the Bible. Jesus' healing touch was a large part of his ministry. Wherever Jesus went, people were pressing in on him, trying to touch him. Luke tells us that on one occasion, "the people all tried to touch him, because power was coming from him and healing them all."[19]

The medicinal effects of touch have been well-established over the centuries. *Life* Magazine reported in a 1997 article that the sense of touch is the first to develop in babies still in the womb and the last to fade as we die. Massage has been shown to lower stress hormones, reduce the heart rate and lower blood pressure, among other therapeutic effects. Premature babies who are lovingly touched and massaged in their incubators by hospital personnel gain weight 47 percent faster than babies who don't receive this special attention.[20] Americans are far less touchy-feely than people of other cultures. Studies have shown that in France, for example, where parents and children allegedly touch each other three times more frequently than their American counterparts, children are less aggressive.[21] Cultural and social factors aside, most of us are still far too touch-deprived. If I were to issue a prescription for the loved ones of depressed patients, it would include "a minimum of 10 hugs per day." It's good preventive medicine, too.

Never underestimate the healing power in both your prayer and your touch for a loved one who is suffering emotionally. You have been empowered by the Holy Spirit to aid in this kind of healing, whether you realize it or not. Ever since the day of Pentecost, when Christ's disciples were first empowered, this healing spirit has been available to all who believe in Jesus. Don't be afraid to use it. And remember, you can pray for yourself. There is no set formula for healing or coping prayer. Research has shown that simple, nonspecific prayers such as "Thy will be done" can be just as effective as detailed petitions. Prayer is not complicated. It's just making contact with God and letting Him, through your faith, do the work of healing. This is what the phrase "Let go and let God" is all about. Believe me, He doesn't need you to tell Him how to do His job. He does expect to be asked, however.

Herbert Vander Lugt, one of the writers for *Our Daily Bread*, has said, "I'm distressed that so many sermons and books today are exclusively devoted to techniques on how to help people cope successfully with life's pains, problems and struggles. ... But without teaching people the great biblical truths of God, His power, His sovereignty, His grace and His salvation through Christ, they get no help in building a solid spiritual foundation for their lives. ... The first step in solving any problem is to make sure we have a right relationship with God, and then seek His wisdom."[22] We can't be afraid of "tough love," either the giving or the receiving.

A similar sentiment was expressed by a Catholic priest who wrote to Dr. Laura Schlessinger:

> Some time ago I began to realize that I was not always serving people as well as I could. ... It is eas-

ier to keep silent under the guise of compassion than to speak the truth that people need to hear, so that they might free themselves with God's help from the self-imposed burdens that bring so much sadness and misery to their own lives and to the lives of other people. This umbrella of false compassion can also protect you from having to look too closely at your own faults. ... I think too often today when people come to a priest seeking advice, he may not want to 'add to their burden' or 'make then feel guilty,' or perhaps it is more important for him to be seen as a kind, caring sort of guy. So he leaves individuals without a challenge, without applying God's law, and without any real tools to improve their lives.[23]

So many people who shy away from Judeo-Christian principles, and likewise, from seeking biblical solutions to their problems, consider God's wisdom a thing not to be grasped. God in the Old Testament through the prophet Isaiah said, "I live in a high and holy place, but also with him who is contrite and lowly in spirit. ..."[24]

Perhaps you've heard the story of the little girl who stood in front of the bathroom mirror peering into her mouth with a flashlight and asking repeatedly, "Are you there? Are you there?" in hopes of getting an immediate response from God. Since early childhood, many of us have been assured by loving parents or Sunday School teachers that God lives in our hearts. As adults, we could use more of that childlike faith when it comes to dealing with adult problems. In fact, because many cases of depression and other mental illnesses have their roots in childhood, traveling back in time through our memories to these innocent, vulnerable days can have a therapeutic effect on us. If this can be accomplished through healing prayer or therapy, so much the better.

When several generations in a family spend time together, such as during weddings, funerals, holidays or family reunions, the memories shared bond each member of that family more tightly and remind one and all of the unique history they have written together. Even when we can't be together, we can remember and celebrate this bond every time we look at those snapshots or home videos or reread a letter. They're priceless treasures that sustain us through the years. Pain and sorrow are more easily borne in the company of our loved ones.

As we are told in the book of Ecclesiastes, "To everything there is a season, and a time to every purpose under the heaven: A time to be born, and a time to die; a time to plant and a time to pluck up that which is planted; A time to kill, and a time to heal; a time to break down, and a time to build up; a time to weep, and a time to laugh; a time to mourn, and a time to dance. ... He hath made everything beautiful in his time."[25] Despair may have its place in our lives, but only for a time, and only to force us to look up. Are we, then, to view endless despair as sin, something which ultimately separates us from God? Despite the clearly established biological component of my illness, I'm convinced that part of my suffering came from willful rebellion against God which was really no more than a prolonged, childish temper tantrum. My own journaling and clear recollections of my thoughts can lead me to no other conclusion. I needed to grow up.

It's interesting to read in the book of Isaiah what God's views toward rebellion, and likewise, toward reconciliation are:

> "I will not accuse forever,
> nor will I always be angry;
> I have seen his ways, but I will heal him;
> I will guide him and restore comfort to him. ..."
> But the wicked are like the tossing sea,
> which cannot rest, whose waves cast up mire
> and mud. "There is no peace," says my God,
> "for the wicked."[26]

Does that not sound like a perfect metaphor for the hell of depression and anxiety: "the tossing sea" that "cannot rest?" That's not to imply that your depression necessarily comes from wickedness (sin), but it does often follow the lack of reconciliation with God. If that is you, and nothing else has worked, then perhaps you're being asked to examine your relationship with God. C.S. Lewis wrote in *Mere Christianity,*

"[God] is the source from which all your reasoning power comes. You could not be right and He wrong any more than a stream can rise higher than its own source."[27] Insightful words. This book will only partially help you until you truly understand that statement. All the loving people in the world cannot surpass the love God has for you or set you on the right course without ultimately leading you to Him and His peace.

The most important epiphany you will ever experience is the moment when you realize you are doomed to failure or destruction unless God alone rescues you.

Seven

The value of marriage is not that adults produce children, but that children produce adults.

Peter De Vries

~~~~~~~~~~~~

Words Of Love And Healing

To know me is also to know my mother and father. You've met them in these pages. It has never been my purpose to indict either of them for any wrongdoing, intentional or unintentional. I hope I have lived up to my mother's assessment of this book as it was being written: "You haven't said anything that isn't true and you have handled it gently." I love my parents very much and owe much appreciation to them for their gifts to me. I never expected them to be perfect, as I hope they never expected me to be.

Perhaps the most appropriate way to illustrate my relationship with my parents and to honor the bond between us is to share some letters that have been written over the years. These letters, and many that I have written, are a part of my family history book, an extended journal. The fabric of our lives is woven throughout these written words. I hope the art of letter writing never dies. Somehow, neither Hallmark nor e-mail capture the same heart-felt emotion as a handwritten letter. Sometimes, we need to have a reaffirmation of our relationships. This I have accomplished by rereading these letters many times. I have discovered that some of the perceptions I had of my parents were incorrect. They deserve an opportunity to speak for themselves. I'll begin with my dad. The earliest letters I have are more than 23 years old, going back to the first time I was away from home in Austria after graduating from college. Mom was in Germany and Dad was back in Virginia. Dad was going through some significant changes as he had begun his alcoholism recovery program through a state hospital and Alcoholics Anonymous. Occasionally, he would bare his soul to me, sometimes becoming quite philosophical. Notice how many different ways he signs his letters. The fact that he could never call himself "Daddy" is an indication of how much he despised his early years of parenting. I don't think he felt he deserved that title. No matter. I've never stopped calling him Daddy:

February 2, 1977
Dear Debbie,

I received your letter the other day and was real glad to hear from you. I'm also happy to know that you are doing well.

I got moved into my own apartment here last week. It's quite nice. The doctor and counselor at the D.A.S. thought I should leave the Full Circle House and get a place of my own. I'm very content now and I live just one day at a time. That is the way I work at my sobriety. It feels nice to have almost eight months of that and to lose my physical sickness and mental anguish and torment that alcohol dependency had brought on — the remorse and resentments, guilt and jealousy, etc. ...

I think of Florida and still miss it at times. I'd like to return to live there permanently. I feel now, should I return and refrain from alcohol, things would be much different. The other times, I used it as a geographical escape which never works for an alcoholic wanting to stay on the "wet" side. ...

I must now bring this letter to a close wishing you in the future happy and pleasant, content days.

Love,
Your father

March 8, 1977
Dear Debbie,

Good morning, Debbie. How are things in Austria? Here in Virginia spring is just around the corner. The robins have

returned from Florida. That is a good sign. I'm still sober going toward the tenth month. I used to stand before the judge getting my time from alcohol abuse. Now I help him here in Honor Court talking to other alcoholics and persons with drinking problems. I spoke there last Wednesday night. It gave me great satisfaction. ...
Yesterday was a rough day on the job, as most days are. I think most of this is my fault since I'm too much a perfectionist. That can be bad in a lot of respects. Then, too, I think a little paranoia is good. Some fears are blessings in disguise. ...
I have stayed sober since I left to be on my own. Thank the God of my understanding, He has done it for me. Not all as I've had to help myself a lot. It's true God helps those who help themselves. But sometimes a man wishes he had never grown up and left the sandbox. ...
We have a book to write, you and I. Together, we can do it. I feel people can be miles apart and communicate, like the porpoises at sea.
So now in closing let me say I think God has been paving the way to my goal as fast as He can lay the asphalt. I must take it a might easier and let time work it out. Oh, and how I push against the tide of time and buck every wave until my poor ship is torn and battered. ...
Let's pray for a brighter tomorrow

Honestly written,
Your father

The next letters I have from my dad were written after I left the Marine Corps and came to California. I had just gone through my divorce.

May 21, 1981
Dear Debbie,
Now that the clouds of life have cleared a bit, I'll write a few lines to you. May I first say I hope this letter finds you happy and content and in perfect serenity.
We laid your Grandmother Effie to rest on Monday. She passed on to eternity the same month as your Grandfather

Hebron at approximately the same hour in the morning as he. I arose from my bed on that morning at that exact time to start my duties for the day. ... She had a lovely funeral. ... Rev. Crady gave the congregation in his sermon a message of high praise for her. ... Your grandfather is being removed from the farm to rest eternally beside her. ...

We have nothing to do with choosing who our parents will be, our birthday or our day of death. But the rest in life is of our choosing. I have to think of what Davy Crockett said: "Be sure you're right and then go ahead."

I enjoyed our lunch and short time we spent together and talked in March. I wish it could have been longer. ...

I would like to say in closing may the good Lord bless and keep you until we meet again.

Love,
Father

June 21, 1981

Dear Debbie,

Thanks for your nice letter. At least it shows you care. ... I enjoy the time I give volunteering in alcoholism counseling. It also helps me.

Last Sunday, I got an A.K.C. registered beagle pup from a guy in Lynchburg who went to college with your brother, Harold Jr. I hope to get back into rabbit hunting. Remember the pups in the shop and the time you let one fall onto the floor and thought you had killed it and ran to the house?

Yes, Debbie, I hit the bottom, but the longer I stay in sobriety the more I pick up of the things I lost. I'm glad you have both feet on the ground. It's true every tub has to stand on its own bottom.

For the sake of yourself and God, never have to lean on a crutch to cope with the realities of life.

I'll sign with best of luck to you and Russ.

Love,
Father

January 15, 1982
Dear Debbie and Russ,
God has laid upon my heart to write this letter to you. First, let me say I think Russ is a swell person, but you must understand that God does not make any mistakes. He brought the two of you together for a purpose.
You must understand your man at all times, Debbie. Not only that, but you must believe in him. ... Put far from you negative thoughts and actions. ...
Jesus knew the way He must go and follow in His father's business. That is why He had to put the Devil behind Him and not have him or his likeness in front of Him to hamper his every move or task. ... The evil forces will surround you to stop a move that you want to make if the intent is positive or for good. However, if the move is negative or for evil, the road to hell will open wide. ...
You two can accomplish so much together and good for God and the Lord. Always love your Lord, Debbie. He is beside you, but He wants you to love Him and trust Him. Put your arms around Him now. ...
I myself and my angels with the help of the Almighty God are back on the front lines ready for battle once more, but this time we have God on our side. He will give the orders. We will be His actors on the stage of life. ...
Pray every day. God loves you and so do I. The Lord must love Russ or he wouldn't have married you.

Love,
Father

December 8, 1985
Dear Debbie,
Sorry I haven't answered your letter sooner, but as usual, I've been busy with this and that. ...
On December, hunting season opens for primitive weapons. I got a 45 cal. percussion black powder Kentucky rifle kit and put it together. It is very accurate. I'm really looking forward to hunting with it. ... I really enjoyed putting it together as a hobby. Sometimes I feel like I'm ready to be put

out to pasture, then somehow I get a new surge again. But just to be in the forest again with nature around me has brought back so many memories of days gone by. I picture many past hunts — that mountain I climbed at Sherando — and once again think, can I still do it? The challenge to do it draws closer every day. Once again, I'll try it. That is life. Always keep another mountain to climb as one can never climb them all.

I'm pleased to learn you and Russ are expecting. I hope it is a boy. I think when one's daughter is expecting, it's a bit more exciting than a son sowing, or at least that is how I feel

I wish you both a Merry Christmas and a happy new year.

Sincerely with love,
Harold Sr.

August 23, 1986

Dear Russ and Debbie,

I've enjoyed looking at the pictures of my granddaughter. She is a fine baby. ... I haven't been back long from the church. Julie was married to Tom today. I gave her away. Rev. Crady performed the ceremony. ...

I only wish I could have given you away in marriage, but fate didn't let that happen. Then, during my days of alcohol abuse, time flew so quickly and all of you were grown but Jeff, and even he was far away.

Sometimes we wonder why we do things and wonder if we made the right turns. And then looking back, we wonder how many things are predestined. Oh well, call it what you may. What will be will be, I guess. ...

I managed to take a few days of vacation at Williamsburg last week. ... Jamestown is a lot different than when I took you children. More has been added. I wonder if Harold Jr. still has that rusty spike I found in front of the church there. As I stood in front of it this time, that is the first thing that came to mind. Oh well, so much for bygones. ...

Well, keep me posted on the baby's progress and write whenever you can. Love you both.

Sincerely,
Harold Sr.

I believe those letters speak for themselves. Needless to say, my dad's recovery inspired me with much hope to find my way back from the darkness of depression. That my father still felt the necessity to give me advice has been precious to me. I wish I had taken some of that advice more to heart.

Now we come to my mom. She also corresponded with me when I was in Austria, but we didn't see the need for much philosophizing then. Some of her most significant letters came during the period when I was facing great struggles in the latter days of my Marine Corps career. I kept much of my family at arm's length for a while as I sorted things out for myself. I don't have any letters from my dad during that time. He was unsure of what was happening. Reading these letters reminds me that everything is temporal. There will be some good and bad in every age, but always there will be some blessing to reflect upon.

May 4, 1980
Dear Debbie,

A month has passed and I haven't heard a word from you. I have three letters from (your husband) and one from his mother, but Debbie, I want to hear from you how you are doing! Don't shut me out, Debbie! ... We are a close family and are concerned about your well-being. ... We are your family, and though we may not approve, we still love you and care about you. You must know us well enough to understand that.

If you have irresolvable differences, then so be it. I have my own theories about a lasting relationship between you and Russ, but you are the one who must live with your decision. I do want you to keep in mind the fact that you may have difficulty loving any one man because you were denied a father's love as a child. ...

Debbie, you are my only daughter and it hurts to think you are facing problems with values. ... We all hurt for you, so please don't shut us out of your life. That is like compounding everything else. Please write soon.

Love,
Mom

August 24, 1980
Dear Debbie,
 Your letter came yesterday. I was really glad to hear from you. I'm very concerned that this "fiasco" is still dragging on. I really hope and pray that the scars will soon go away. ...
 Debbie, I'm really concerned since you have no family nearby that you maintain some contact with a friend. ...
 Hang in there and remember that though I don't understand all that has taken place, (your husband) has succeeded in doing one thing he didn't really aim to do. He had drawn us much closer together rather than drive us apart. ...
 Please write often as I am very concerned over you.

Much love,
Mom

November 8, 1980
Dear Debbie,
 This makes the second letter I've started. What I say just doesn't seem to sound right and I'm afraid you'll read into what I say. You have enough problems now without my adding to them. You need understanding, love and prayer, perhaps like you have never needed it before. ...
 I sure hope that by the time this letter reaches you, your troubles are over. I'm praying that you might consider getting away from everyone involved there and rediscovering yourself as an individual. ...
 Whatever the outcome, Debbie, you'll need faith in yourself and faith that God will see you through, it you let Him. ...
 Lord knows, I love you and want you to have a good life, but I fear that your choices have temporarily gotten in the way. Lord help you to choose wisely from this point on, or else be able to accept the consequences if you don't. It's certainly a helpless feeling when you just wait and wait for a whole complicated situation to unravel. I've asked myself a million times, Why? ...
 Please write SOON.

Love,
Mom

December 3, 1980
Dear Debbie,

Thanks so much for your letter and clippings. I must say I was shocked to see the details in print, but glad to know you feel comfortable in sharing your dilemma with me. I am certainly doubling my prayer efforts and concern that all will end soon and you'll know what adjustments need to be made in order to go on with your life, without too many scars. Many times I have thought how good my hindsight is — if only I could have seen that beforehand. Unfortunately, or maybe even sometimes fortunately, we only learn some things by actual experience. I'm sure you'll accept the responsibility of your choices the same as I have done and move on from there. ...

One wants the best for her children. Their problems become magnified when they reach you. Can't explain it, but believe me, it's so! I have had to accept, adapt my views and roll with each situation. And yet, how thankful I am for a Lord to help me shoulder each problem as it arises. ...

Lots of love,
Mom

February 1, 1981
Dear Debbie,

I can't believe I've taken so long to answer your beautiful, long letter. ... I can only assume that your case remains unresolved since I didn't get a follow-up letter or a phone call. ...

I do believe this is the worst year I have had since your dad was having all his problems. I really thought all major heartaches were behind me. If the Lord metes out heartaches according to how much He loves you, I must surely be loved.

I'm so sorry I didn't write to you my real gut feeling about your marriage. I wanted to say, Debbie, I know it's wrong. I didn't, so I must write my gut feeling now. ... Russ may be the one for you, but you must back off to know for sure. It's so hard to write this in a letter for fear you'll misinterpret what I'm trying to say. ... Please try to understand the hurt when your children (even if they're grown) are having problems. You can't "kiss it away" like you did when they were little.

You just have to trust and have faith that they rely on God's help in their daily lives. Please get on your knees and pray, Debbie, for guidance and wisdom in making your next choice. Don't try to do it alone.

I'll be anxiously waiting for your next letter. Remember I love you and I am concerned.

Lots of love,
Mom

April 17, 1981
Dear Debbie,

I was so glad to get your letters and the picture and to know that you are settled in, though temporarily, in California. I really do like the picture of you and Russ. Jeff was particularly impressed by the medals and wants to know what each one is.

Glad you enjoyed the trip across country and that you could ski. Also glad you could meet Russ' family. ...

As I have prayed for each of you children this year, I feel that I, too, have become a different person. I am sending you a copy of the prayer calendar from church. Notice that you are on the 10th and we're on the 16th. ...

I am thankful most of all that you have almost made it through your rough ordeal. I guess you feel you have made it through now that you've left North Carolina. My prayers, hopes and desires are for smooth sailing ahead, or at least the ability to cope with each situation as it arises. I think each one of you kids, as you have pointed out numerous times, certainly have had enough preparation for coping with varied situations. ...

When I think that 27 years ago, I was anxiously waiting and hoping you'd be a little girl, it makes me wish I could be there to celebrate your birthday with you. You'll know I'm thinking of you all day long — not only then, but every morning and night of every day when I ask God to watch over each of you. Though we had rough times during those years when you kids were growing up, I feel that God has blessed us far beyond any bad experiences we may have had temporarily. How thankful I am for each of you and your accomplishments. ...

Russ made a favorable impression on Harold Jr. I like his

looks in the picture. Even though I can't say I approve of your beginning relationship, I'm certainly not perfect either. We have all made mistakes and must cope and move from there. All my good wishes for the best that life has to offer.

Lots of love,
Mom

I'll fast-forward about six years to a letter I received from my mom after I'd announced we were expecting our second child. Because we lived so far apart for more than 20 years, we relied on letters and, of course, phone calls to communicate many times. Just this year, I've come back to my childhood home where many family members still reside. I miss those letters, to tell the truth. I have loved my mom's optimism and practical prescriptions for life's ailments, and she knows I will attempt to reign her in when she drifts toward any pessimism. I know she has left her indelible imprint on me. Coincidentally, we both spent about the same amount of time (17-18 years) living far away from "home." Those years broadened our horizons in similar ways. Even though we don't always agree, my mom is my friend.

March 25, 1987
Dear Debbie, Russ and Jennifer,
    I've been thinking about you folks, especially since the phone call with the big news! Even though you are probably still in the "mixed blessings" mode, remember all things work together for good, to those who love the Lord. God sees the total picture in the divine plan and parenting is certainly a part of family life, a big part. ...
    Being 16 months apart, Jennifer and the new baby will be very close to each other. Sibling rivalry should be minimal. ... If the new baby arrives on my birthday, that will be special in itself!
    By the time this letter arrives, you should have received another package. ... Please forgive me if I'm indulging that beautiful baby! ...
    Today is Granddaddy Mays' birthday (120th) and he

always said, "Give me the roses while I live." That's my philosophy, too. I was able to do so few material things for you kids while you were growing up. The Lord blessed us in so many ways, though, and He is blessing me in other ways at present so that I can share a little extra with each of you now. Maybe it's better this way because if I had been blessed with more money when you kids were growing up, I probably would have been an indulgent mom! Result — spoiled children. I'll take the unspoiled variety and the indulging later from Grandma!

Everybody is going in so many different directions, I can hardly keep up. ... The Lord seems to be blessing everybody. That doesn't mean that we can rest on our laurels as there are always those little situations that could gnaw away at our core of being — we just need to put them into perspective and forge on. ...

Looking forward to your next letter.

Love you all,
Mom, Lourine,
Grandma "M"

I'd like to honor my mother by sharing a poem she wrote when I was a little girl and sent to me in a letter several years ago. I had never seen it before then. Though it may have been written for my brothers and me while we were babes, I take great comfort in reading it today. I've learned in recent years that Mom wrote poetry to help her cope with tough situations.

FAIL ME NOT

Oh, please do help me, said a little child,
My steps are wobbly, the path I humbly tread;
And tiny feet grow weary, yet it's day
with unapparent night time still ahead.
Oh, guide me through the jungle lest I fall,
The way is narrow and I stumble so,
That you must take my hand and lead me on
to steady steps on firmer ground below.

I pray for help and guidance while 'tis day
Oh, won't you raise a prayer to Heaven above?
A little child requested me in faith.
And I responded, "YES," for God is love,
Who reaches down in his abiding grace
to lead us both to safety, so don't fall;
Together we may conquer many paths
And win eternal life — that is God's call.

Lourine M. Massie
1962

Eight

Truth hurts — not the searching after; the running from!
John Eyberg

~~~~~~~~~~~~

I've Got To Be Me, But Who Am I?

There are few joys that can compare with the feeling of being released from a long, emotional illness, or any illness, for that matter. I remained elated for months after realizing that my medication had successfully abated my depressive episodes. Even though my doctor felt that I might have a 50 percent chance of relapsing into depression without the medication, I had no worries. I decided to live in the other 50 percent realm. I chose that as my reality. Nevertheless, I was prepared to take Desyrel for the rest of my life, if it became necessary. Robert Louis Stevenson, who suffered from consumption much of his life, once said, "I have not let the medicine bottle on my mantle become the limit to my vision." Fortunately, for me there were barely any unpleasant side effects. In fact, the only side effect to speak of was a good one — I was thinner, due either to a changed metabolism or a reduced appetite. This was a welcome change from the increased appetite and resulting weight gain I had experienced on Elavil.

Because I was feeling so healthy, I was totally unprepared for the backlash that awaited me. It hit me with no warning and turned my world upside down. Russ and I were both left wondering whether it might have been more desirable to revert back to the depressive episodes. At least that was an old, familiar pain.

In order for me to describe the challenges I faced, it is necessary for me to revisit some of my past. I had not considered myself particularly outgoing during my youth. In fact, I was a painfully shy child in school. As I approached adulthood, I gradually began to come out of my shell. The greatest boost to my self-confidence came during my years in the Marine Corps. There, I honed my self-sufficiency and leadership skills, something I think my mother had tried to teach me all my life. When I was at the peak of my short-lived career, I fell from grace and lost my chief means for achieving recognition and respect as a result of the disciplinary actions taken against me. It was Russ who pointed out to me years later that I was still in need of that recognition.

Each episode of depression I experienced took me back further into a childlike state of fear and uncertainty. It was painful to remember where I had been at the pinnacle of my Marine Corps career and to realize where I had regressed. When I was finally free from depression, I wasted little time in seeking to regain my former status. It seemed I couldn't do enough fast enough. Most of my efforts went into pursuing an interest in music that had always been there, but had been squelched by my negativity. Now, nothing seemed impossible. The world was wide open to me, and I found myself wanting to do everything that I previously couldn't. I felt reborn in a dramatic way. I began to like myself.

I also found I had a strong desire to build friendships with other people. The lack of meaningful friendships had been a frustrating part of my former life. It had been difficult for me to let others get very close. Now, it seemed almost essential that I have close friends. All this pursuit of outside interests began to put a strain on my marriage. I was so different from before that Russ had a hard time coping with my needs. We seemed to be at odds frequently, our priorities clashing most of the time. I failed to see at first how selfish I was becoming. Before I knew it, we were in the midst of enormous conflict. I wanted to challenge Russ on practically everything. It seemed we argued incessantly. I was still somewhat out of control, only at the opposite end of the spectrum now. I wanted Russ to approach life as enthusiastically as I was. In my view, he wasn't living up to his potential. Now that I had recovered, I set out to "fix"

Russ, who of course needed time to recover from all those years of caring for me. I was rushing ahead of him. We needed balancing desperately.

It isn't difficult to see how the stage was set for me to seek an outside pressure-relief valve. With my chaste record already blotted by past events, I suppose I felt less guilt in seeking solace outside my marriage. Past pain and my rediscovered faith had kept me from even considering being unfaithful to this point. In my misguided quest for self-realization (how I hate that word!), I took one fateful step too far. If I thought the crisis depression brought to our marriage was severe, I was about to see it overshadowed by a crisis far more severe — infidelity.

The most difficult quality of a marriage to regain once it is lost is trust. I willfully walked away from my first marriage having never really built a foundation. I didn't want to go back. But it was different this time. Deep down, I couldn't fail at marriage again. Yet, I was mired to the hip in that most treacherous of quagmires and was sinking fast. Few marriages can survive this trauma. Our union of 10 years was tested to its limits, but I didn't want it to end. I couldn't bear losing Russ. I knew he was God's gift to me, and it is solely by God's grace that Russ and I were able to rebuild our marriage. Restoring a marriage whose vows have been tarnished takes more patience and prayer than most people think is humanly possible. And it takes time. The humility required of me to accept my husband's forgiveness brought me to my knees. The course of our marriage is forever changed. Like Adam and Eve in the garden, we lost the pristine sanctity of our union and had to labor at our relationship like never before. But God is a god of love. His chief business is unity. If we didn't believe He wanted to restore our marriage, we could never have taken the first step toward reconciliation. The positive aspect of a marriage that has rebounded from the brink of destruction is that both partners appreciate each other more and develop a keener sense of outside intrusions from that point on.

In order to fully explain the nature of my relationship with Russ, I must again digress back to my years as a single and review the events that led up to our eventual union.

I had dated a high school sweetheart for several years,

beginning with my senior year in high school. For a while, we believed we would marry, but knew we would have to wait until we both finished college because he had chosen to attend a military academy, and marriage was prohibited for him. He was 500 miles away, however, and the distance had put quite a strain on our relationship. By mid-college, it started going downhill, fast. In my senior year, he became engaged to another girl. I was informed in a letter, and needless to say, was devastated. I couldn't see then that he was not the man for me. I had already forgiven him once for past indiscretions. After all, we weren't married. But I had needed him desperately. The feelings of betrayal and rejection coupled with my confusion over what I wanted to do with my life sent me into a tailspin, which spawned another traumatic event and a stillborn relationship. I was confused and in great pain. My mom was preparing to go overseas to Germany to embark on a teaching career. I had been offered a position as a journalist with a small-town newspaper. I decided instead to accompany my mom to Germany. So great was my desire to escape as far away as I could from the site of my misery, that I sold my Volkswagen for $500, the cost of a one-way airline ticket to Frankfurt. I didn't even want to think about coming home.

For the next few months, I nursed my wounds. I spent time trying to analyze myself and figure out how I might have contributed to my broken relationship. I had been somewhat clingy and perhaps too hasty in desiring matrimony. In fact, I had desperately wanted to be married. Apparently, desperate women aren't too attractive to men. I couldn't see then that I had a huge hole in my heart, left over from childhood. I was trying to fill it the only way I knew how. I later learned that this void was responsible for my depression in many ways. I had some mistaken impressions about myself in my younger years. My unhappy childhood had left me vulnerable and in great need of love. My quest for the love that I perceived would make me whole took me on a painful journey, and sometimes to unhealthy places. I became well-acquainted with rejection, the most significant of which was self-rejection. I hated who I thought I was.

After my European experience was over, I came back to the

States, determined to embark on a career as a military officer. I was still looking for some stability in my life. I thought the armed services would provide that, and I was right. But what a bittersweet time it would prove to be! I chose the toughest road — the Marine Corps. They delivered on their promise: it was no rose garden. I grew up a lot in the Marines. Those years largely shaped who I am today.

As it turned out, I ended up being stationed at Camp Lejeune, North Carolina when my nine months of officer training were over, in the same office with Russ Thurman. (I've often noted with amusement that the Marine Corps considers nine months the proper gestation period required to "birth" an officer). There I was, a baby-faced lieutenant with "butter bars" on my collar, out in the real Fleet Marine Force for the first time. As if the road ahead weren't already tough enough, I had a new lieutenant husband walking it with me. I'd had my lovely, storybook wedding, complete with arched swords. But that's where the fairy tale ended.

I'm not proud of the way in which I went about dissolving my marriage, but I was young and I felt as if that relationship betrayed everything about me. Even so, Russ and I fell under God's judgment as revealed in Proverbs:

> But a man [or woman] who commits adultery lacks judgment; whoever does so destroys himself. ... and his shame will never be wiped away.[1]

I wonder how many people suffer the indignation of depression which results from choosing to pursue an adulterous relationship. All parties are usually emotionally devastated. This curse can follow you for a long time — forever, in fact, if we're to believe the verses above. Perhaps that's why I so easily chose that path a second time.

My mom tried to convince me to take time away, completely to myself, but I would have none of that. I might have been better off had I taken her advice because Russ would have waited for me. But I had never felt more complete that I did with Russ, and being a stubborn individual, I clung to him, somehow sensing that God just might have a hand in this relationship. We were married soon after my divorce was final.

Russ and I fought the battle of my depression together for the next 10 years. Little did I know that, even though I felt I had finally found what I had been seeking, I was repressing feelings and issues that I still had to deal with. So was Russ. We both had a trail of broken relationships behind us and had some similar childhood pains, as well. If depression comes from both biological and psychological causes, you may feel better after using antidepressants or other remedies. But, rest assured, unresolved issues will rear their heads again at some point. A spirit that is broken has to be mended.

I was devastated to find that my restlessness and confusion had resurfaced following my recovery from depression. When I finally realized what it was all about, after much counseling and reading, I felt somewhat absolved of guilt over who I was. The guilt I faced over what I did was another matter. I won't detail the moral issues I had to deal with at this point because this was a very private matter, between God and me, but I know others have faced or will face similar struggles. I know because there is nothing new under the sun. Likewise, God knows this and He is the supreme counselor. He understands the most complex of feelings, no matter how odious you may think they are.

The toughest struggle Russ and I ever had to face in our marriage was the period of about two years following my recovery from depression during which I felt very strongly that I had to act on my compulsive urges. If I could go back and relive any part of my life, I would want to have the chance to wipe the slate clean during that part of our marriage and undo the foolish acts I committed in the name of self-actualization. I am still doing penance, in a sense, for those transgressions. I knew Russ would never have deserted me during the years of my illness. He truly believed he had married me for better or worse, in sickness and in health. But my unfaithfulness was very nearly the undoing of our marriage. If I view my healing from the despair of depression as a miracle, then it is almost inconceivable to think of the great compassion God must have had for me in restoring our marriage following my senseless acts of treason. He had to change two hearts, not just one.

God actively used whatever means He could to bring me

back under His protection and love during this time. There were incredible interventions that could only be viewed as divine. After I realized that God was not going to let me wander any further off the path He had established for me, I actually began to pray for His interventions. I asked Him to protect me from my own foolishness, no matter what the cost. He answered those prayers. Again, I felt I had a thorn in the flesh to contend with. Naturally, I prayed for it to be removed, but that happened only in part. It was grace, once again, that I had to receive, in order to overcome this new battle. Today, I'm in the final stages of that healing process. I've learned it doesn't come about overnight, but I've stayed on course, and God has been faithful.

Owning up to rebellion in your life can be a bitter pill to swallow, but rebellion against God and my husband is the only way I can describe my attitude and actions during that time. "Why?" I have asked myself time and time again. I didn't think myself capable of such selfishness. But I am a product of this fallen world, as all human beings are, and sin is both ugly and selfish.

God created us with a desire to have us willingly come to Him and acknowledge Him as the divine source of all that we are. But He gave us freedom of choice so that our love would be meaningful. I believe we have a number of optional paths which we can pursue, any of which can ultimately lead us to His divine goal for us, His will. Some are shorter, some are longer. God chooses the best path for us, but we don't always listen to His instruction. We can choose to go off in the weeds and wander aimlessly for a while or take the more direct path, which we seldom seem to be inclined to do. God graciously allows for course corrections, but there are land mines in the weeds, and we may end up wounded and limping to our destination.

When the pain of those old "war wounds" reminds me of my past transgressions, I find I can control it with thoughts of gratitude for God's grace in my life. Though many of us have read it in the Bible at some point and it makes for great devotional reading, the concept of giving praise in our trials is a hard one to grasp and actually practice. Yet, I have found that in doing so, I have gained more peace and inner strength. It was James, the half-brother of Jesus, who said, "Consider it pure joy, my brothers, whenever you face trials of many kinds, because you know that the testing of your faith develops perseverance."[2]

Another well-known treatise on trials appears in Paul's epistle to the Romans: "But we also rejoice in our sufferings, because we know that suffering produces perseverance; perseverance, character; and character, hope."[3] An attitude of gratitude, even for our pain, will take us a long way toward inner healing, if we will let it. Remember, it's our thinking we are asked to change when we face adversity, not our feelings. We can't *feel* our way out of depression, but we can *think* our way out of it in many cases. What James and Paul are telling us is to stay in the fight, no matter how much we feel like quitting.

I stopped trying to control my undesirable feelings, which of course, did not all go away. I received the strength and the patience to face them and deal with them. This was a psychological reality. Something that takes many years to develop does not disappear overnight. I found I had to take a deep breath and let each wave of pain crash over me as I swam out in the deep waters where only God was my life preserver. Eventually, the sea became calmer and I became a stronger swimmer. Russ and I both feel that our former brokenness is our strength today. Yes, it has been an incredibly painful ordeal, but we have grown tremendously from it. I hope that our experiences can help others who also are engaged in this struggle. We must all remember that, although we react with childish reflexes to some situations in adulthood, we are mature enough to accept adult responsibility for our choices. Sometimes, we just need to choose to grow up fully.

One of the hardest, but most helpful things I did in dealing with my marital struggles was to confide in a trusted friend. I had learned to do this through my battles to overcome depression. In opening up with a friend I felt safe with, I developed a relationship of accountability. I must caution anyone seeking this avenue to make sure that the friend is a mature, trusted, nonjudgmental friend — a "native," as Bernie Siegel would say. I tried this kind of open dialogue with another close friend, but found out that she was still working through some past struggles of her own. This confiding could have been unhealthy had I allowed it to continue. Some people may only be able to have this kind of open, honest relationship with a professional counselor. I had that, too, fortunately. A good friend who loves unconditionally is hard, but not impossible, to find. I recently had the occasion to thank my friend for her willingness to listen to me. Having someone who knows you inside and out and yet still loves you is truly one of life's greatest blessings.

In my counseling to overcome this problem, I came to realize how my depression had been related to my early developmental needs more than I cared to admit. I had tried hard to repress those misplaced feelings, not being able to understand them for many years. Isn't it ironic that, just at the peak of my celebration in recovery from depression, that old monster I had buried should return with a vengeance? When we stop to celebrate a spiritual victory, we often forget that Satan is lurking about, waiting to remind us of other weaknesses. Russ has said to me that I became a very self-centered person during this struggle. I know he is right. I felt as if I had a right to explore and know this side of me — that somehow, I would come full circle and be complete if I did. Did Satan subtly convince me of that? Nothing else seemed to matter at the time. It took a while to deal with the guilt I felt, but today I take a realistic view of why it happened. I know that is not who I am or who God created me to be. Nor do I have any desire to be that person ever again.

I developed a trusting relationship for about a year with a Christian therapist who understood my unique struggles — Diane Eller-Boyko, a licensed clinical social worker. Diane understood me like no one else could. In all my previous relationships with counselors, I had never dealt with the real heart of my problems. She was able to shed light on what my struggle was all about. We talked a lot about my relationship with my parents, particularly with my mom. Although I'm sure our relationship had started out early in my life as a bond of protective love and maternal nurturing, my perception was that it was short-circuited somewhere along the way. For some reason, I wasn't being mothered in the way in which I needed to be. My guess is that this happened when my mom became too distracted by my dad's drinking problem. She could not sustain the superhuman effort required to nurture us all.

Diane's analysis of my situation is this:

> If people are willing to look at the dynamics of their past, at their socialization or where they came from, particularly in relationships with parents, they can come to grips with nurturing issues. You had some issues with your mother [and of course, with my father] which created some type of defensive wall that said "this is not safe." She had some emotional instability and maybe wasn't particularly nurturing because of her own emotional distractions. There has to be an availability, a trusting that if I go to this source, they will be there for me. And as we go and seek them out and find that they are not available any more, we stop going there. A defensive detachment starts to happen.

Diane describes this kind of emotional quest from both a psychodynamic and a Christian viewpoint. As Christians, she says, "our souls are panting after something because of our natural fallen state. We're naturally going to be prone to move in the direction that gives us some kind of wholeness and well-being." She calls this a "hungering heart" or "hole in the heart." We're all searching, she believes, for something at the soul level. Though the kind of ego gratification I was seeking in attaching to other people, which even included dependent relationships with other maternal figures, often happens when through our normal development, nurturing needs go unmet, not all people form this kind of attachment. Others may become addicted to work, to alcohol or drugs. I needed the kind of approbation and connectedness one can only get from intimate relationships. The good news is that's what godly marriage is all about. Show me a woman who has a healthy marriage along with healthy female friendships, and I'll show you a woman who is whole. That's God's plan. Marriage is also intended to be a cord of three strands, with God being the stronger center strand.

It most assuredly wasn't God's plan for me to go through this struggle. But once I had exercised my free will (and a very strong will at that!) and had become embroiled in this emotional battle, His presence became more real to me. He was there at my greatest time of need and sustained me while I wandered through the desert until I came to the place where I could lay my pain to rest once and for all. The poem entitled "Footprints," which describes how God often carries us when we're too weary to walk, is particularly poignant for me. Putting my past in perspective and feeling totally healthy for the first time in my life has been the result of placing my pain in God's hands. I realize there is no pain too great for God to handle, and my hope for things to come in this life, but even more in the next, is heightened. The pleasures that I have sought in this world will pale next to the glories of eternity.

C.S. Lewis has observed, "Our natural experiences are like penciled lines on flat paper. If our natural experiences vanish in the risen life, they will vanish only as penciled lines vanish from the real landscape; not as a candle flame that is put out, but as a candle flame which becomes invisible because someone has pulled up the blind, thrown open the shutters and let in the blaze of the rising sun."[4]

Nine

> Lord of my love, to whom in vassalage
> Thy merit hath my duty strongly knit,
> To thee I send this written ambassage,
> To witness duty, not to show my wit.
>
> William Shakespeare
> Sonnet 26

~~~~~~~~~~~~

No Greater Love

It is fitting that my husband's own words should appear somewhere in this book. He alone has suffered the relentless hell of the day-to-day existence that marks living with someone suffering from major depression. He lived through the confusion that even my coming out of depression brought into our lives. So many times he has been the calm in the midst of the storm. He was called upon to lay down his life nearly every day as he cared for me. He always put me and my needs first. I look back into our past together and see the many ways that I have loved Russ Thurman. Who this man was and is can best be glimpsed through his own eyes, as he writes about himself and about our love.

There is much that I won't share with the world. I prefer to keep our most sacred memories safe between us where they belong. I have never been able to escape the feeling deep in my soul that, despite the pain and hardships we faced, Russ and I were meant to be together. I have great difficulty even expressing the depth of my feelings for him. Despite its temporary tarnishment, I still consider our marriage a priceless treasure and a gift from God. That God wanted us to stay married was confirmed many times over by His continually bringing us back to Him each time we wandered off course.

As I look back on those turbulent days in the Corps while my career was being prematurely terminated, I no longer have any bitterness. True, those events had a tremendously negative impact on my life. I think of two senior officers in my command at the time. I spoke of them both in the opening chapter of this book. One was my battalion commander, the other was on the commanding general's staff. The latter was a gentle man who knew the Lord and spoke to me lovingly about things eternal. My battalion CO on the other hand was a vindictive man who sneered at our relationship and predicted that Russ would desert me at the first opportunity. I left his office, shaking the sand off my boots, and moved on to a life that I am now happy to own.

Russ' correspondence with me began back in the days when we shared the Marine Corps experience. Military life is a unique existence. I always felt very privileged to be a part of the distinguished Marine Corps "brotherhood" even when I couldn't completely understand it. I worked very hard at earning the respect of my peers. That Russ Thurman, Vietnam veteran, heavily bedecked with medals and held in the highest esteem by privates and generals alike, would even take note of me, much less appreciate me, was almost beyond my comprehension. In the unique, Marine Corps sense of the term, he became my mentor. This was our initial relationship, and it progressed to one of mutual respect. There appeared to be no gender boundaries in the beginning. We were Marine officers, pure and simple.

Gradually, I grew to appreciate Russ at a deeper level. For all his greatness, I sensed a large void in him. It was as though I alone could understand him. I longed to see him happy, realizing that there was little I could do to make it so except in a professional sense. In a society where spouses go off in different directions each day to their respective workplaces, either by choice or necessity, it is inevitable that some version of this story will play itself out in many marriages. Russ and I both derived great satisfaction from working together. The likelihood that we would fall in love didn't occur to us at first. We dubbed ourselves the "A-Team." In a sense, we thought of ourselves as being separated from the masses of mediocrity. Russ was so sensible. He possessed uncanny abilities to think on his feet and we were always pulling off some coup or another. I relished the joy of accomplishing another A-Team victory with him. In some ways, it has been difficult to recreate that kind of relationship since our glory days as Marines, even though we've worked together in other capacities. Nevertheless, the "Golden Times," as we called them, still live on in our memories. Today, we possess something even more precious.

Russ and I discovered early on that we shared an appreciation of Shakespeare. In fact, we each presented the other a special keepsake volume of Shakespeare's verse. Perhaps a fitting introduction to Russ' letters to me is my favorite Shakespearean sonnet (116), second only in its eloquent description of love to Paul's famous epistle to the Corinthians in the New Testament.

> Let me not to the marriage of true minds
> Admit impediments. Love is not Love
> Which alters when it alteration finds,
> Or bends with the remover to remove:
> O, no! It is an ever-fixed mark,
> That looks on tempests and is never shaken;
> It is the star to every wandering bark,
> Whose worth's unknown, although his height
>   be taken.
> Love's not Time's fool, though rosy lips and cheeks
> Within his bending sickle's compass come;
> Love alters not with his brief hours and weeks,
> But bears it out even to the edge of doom.
>   If this be error, and upon me proved,
>   I never writ, nor no man ever loved.

Russ' letters need no commentary from me. They speak an eloquent poetry all their own.

November 22, 1979
Dear Debbie,

I feel like I'm sitting down to write a column. Damn, I'm terrible at writing a letter. But I did want so much to write you. I'm drawn to it, to let you know how I feel. Of course, you already know, but it seems so important to tell you again and again that I Love You. ...

Oh Debbie, do you know, do you really? Please don't ask me why I love you. If I knew that, I could unlock the secret of the universe. And although I've professed such skill, I haven't really mastered that, yet. I will though. I will all because of you. I have grown because of you. I have finally touched life. Yes, it's a long way to Tipperary, but I've been there once — on a Golden Friday when the world stood still and marveled, and laughed and found joy in it all. I tremble thinking there may be even more than the Golden Friday, another step, another move toward a world shared by so few. Not even the greatest of Muses have captured such in the weak tool of words. How do you tell of such? If but I could. Perhaps it shouldn't be captured. Perhaps it's not meant to be shared with the masses. Perhaps it's intended only for those who dare to venture beyond the poet's careless verse. ...

You are indeed a special friend, one I can trust deeply, one who knows Russ Thurman as no one else does — the great weaknesses, the modest strengths, all the faults — but still remains a dear friend. For all this I Love You dearly. Oh that you know this, that you truly feel it, that you trust in it.

Tomorrow's song awaits the Dancers
who dare to step to their own tune.

I Love You,
Russ

December 2, 1979
Dearest Debbie,

I've got it bad — a bad case of the "miss yous." ... Everything I do, you're a part of. Every thought, emotion, hope — you're there, always. ...

Today at church, I prayed for us and lit the three candles. Going to church has helped me a lot. ... The Lord understands, I can feel it.

This morning I was thinking about how I've always said I was scared of the future. That's not true. Yes, I'm scared of failing, but, don't you see, we won't fail. The thought came to me as I was thinking about the song "Old Man River." It's a song that's kept me going when times were tough. See, regardless of how tough life gets, that "Old Man River, he just keeps rolling along." One line in that song really jumped out at me this morning: "Tired of living, but scared of dying." Changed a bit, it goes "Tired of failing, but scared of not trying." There comes a time when everyone has to be counted. I'm standing now! ...

I hear the music and the dance floor is ours. Step to the music, my dear, for the world is ours. I love you, Debbie. I love you dearly.

The moon kissed me softly and warmed me
with its glow when I called your name tonight.

Good Night, Golden Dancer,
Russ

At Sea
March, 1980
Dearest Debbie,

I need so much to reach out and hold you, to pull you close to me, to let you know how much I love you, to tell you of tomorrows, to gather you inside me, to be a part of you, to give strength, to receive the same from you. I love you so much. Your letter means so much to me — every word. It's all there, all that we are, all that we face, all that we can be. ...

The whys, yes, the whys. Why did all this happen? Why would destiny bring us together only to weave such a maze? A test? A challenge? Why would you choose to love me? Why would I, in turn, challenge my very soul to love you? I have few, if any answers. ...

Debbie, you are important. You are someone very special, someone with so very unique qualities, qualities that drew me to you long ago. You have a tenderness that reaches out to soothe, to understand. You are also tough, much more so than you think. You stand well against tough odds. And there's a flame in you, one that cries to be seen, to blaze. You are destined for greatness — greatness on many levels. ...

You spark in me a determination, a drive that is so intense I know I could accomplish anything this world and beyond could offer or demand. ... I love you as a friend. You are truly the best friend I've ever had. I've trusted you with my deepest secrets, my most precious thoughts, my heart. Because of you, I've broken loose from my own bindings, soared in a way I didn't know existed. ... Together we are special — magnificent — in all things. It has been mused over in many ways through the centuries. Sad how poorly the work of the masters; they never knew us. They must cry. ...

My eyes, my heart, my soul are open. I do not peer through rose-colored glasses, drugged by a longing that loneliness demands. To do so would be a hideous betrayal of myself, of you, of us — one deserving of banishment into the far reaches of hell. No, I am not blind. But I am a man, racked with faults, indeed; however, one who has long learned that little matters except the footprints I stand in and those that are ahead. Those behind me are there for all who care to see, to make of what they will, regardless of my intent. I cannot wash them away or gather them up in a futile attempt to rearrange them to the liking of others. Yes, I do want to be liked, to be well-thought of — to be someone special. But too many times in the past, I did what others wanted, what others felt was right, what others expected. And all too often, I disliked myself, hated my stepping to the drummer of others. ...

I stand on my own two feet, knowing full well I cannot live without or apart from others, but at the same time demanding my right to hear my own drummer. Such is the right of all humans, a right bestowed by God. And the Lord and I have had much to talk about of late. In truth, it has been much more difficult to deal with the wronging of God's law than I've revealed. It's not guilt or shame I feel, not really, but rather something else. It all goes very deep inside — to the way I was raised, to a home broken as a child — to promises to myself — to painful memories — to being wronged — to my own tarnishment — violation of personal and sacred vows. And while I fear no man or his laws, I do not stand as staunchly against God. ...

I have long believed the Lord, if not destiny, has presented

the many obstacles as a test, a challenge of my love for you. ...
The Lord must understand, He must. ... In the end, I will make peace with the Lord. He can see into my heart and soul. He knows. ...

I Love You,
Russ

Egypt
November 7, 1981
Dearest Deb,

I've avoided writing this since I've been here — about 24 hours. I guess I just didn't want to convey to you how low I feel. Some of it's because of this exercise, but mostly it's because I'm away from you. I spend all my time thinking about you, about what you're doing, about what we could be doing together. ...

Deb, I'm going through another change in my life — taking another one of my steps. The step has much to do with you. You have changed my life, as I know I've changed yours. I had long ago developed the ability to be on my own, and I liked it that way, or at least I thought. You knew I was lonely — and since that night, you changed my life. ... I love you, my darling. I'm thinking now about our wedding, that beautiful day, the beginning. How beautiful you were, are. It takes this type of separation for me to truly appreciate how precious you are, how special. You, only you can help me unlock the many doors I have closed tight, the doors that lead to the Whispering Leaves and the Golden Times. How so very important you are to me. ...

I Love You,
Russ

November 30, 1981
Dearest Debbie,

Sweet one, I don't know if this will reach you before I get back or even if you'll receive it before we leave for Virginia, but they're taking mail off the ship in the morning, and I just had to write. I've missed writing you, and especially talking to you. I really got spoiled with those telephone calls. ...

I'm sitting in the wardroom lounge of the USS Saipan, in

the same spot where I composed my letters to you during the sailing to England and Norway. Being on this ship has stirred many memories of that time in our lives. ...

I remember our first talk in Norway when you told me of your change of plans, and later when we went for a walk — I was losing you. And when you returned from Germany, again full of doubt. That was the closest I came to dropping it all. But, oh how I loved you, so dearly! You know I look on your doubts during that time with respect. It was hell for you, I know — much of it brought on by me.

But, as I've said before, if you could have easily walked away, without a second thought, then what would that have meant for us, for our marriage? ...

Those were such strange, bittersweet days — they were our agony and ecstasy. And, truth to tell, I'd walk those same footsteps again — time and again — if it meant that I could stand before God and witnesses and exchange rings of gold to bind our lives forever. How I love you. ... Debbie, my wife, thank you for all you have given me. ...

> For all the artists' skills,
> none has captured
> the wondrous beauty
> cast in the candle's glow—
> of you.

Loving You,
Russ

Russ enclosed the following poem in a letter. I believe it also deserves to be included here.

MOMENTS OF MY YEARS

There have been the dark moments of my years,
Struggles against the shattered heart,
    scarred by the tears.
Searching, always wandering, seeking the elusive dream,
Knowing but glimpses of false love,
    grasped from the passing stream.

Dashed and lonely, cast adrift, True Love
    I would not know.
Thus, I accepted a life alone, banished by
    Fate's cruel blow.
Then came a Wind, a Messenger, a Teller of tales so dear.
On Leaves it told of Golden Times, this Whispering Seer.

From before the Dawn of Time She came,
    surrounded by a glow,
Touching me with a Special Love, one only
    Dreamers know.
She gathered me within Her passion,
    opening my secret door,
Singing a song of Lasting Love, that written
    in ancient lore.

But she had to be won, this Lady Fair,
    the Dragon I had to face.
With drawn sword I battled the fire and fury,
    the injustice and disgrace.
She stood beside me, this Warrior Queen,
    to strike awesome blows.
Together we fought the Dragon's Disciples and
    smote the sinister foes.

Today, She caresses with a kiss the scars that I bear,
Within my heart; they're monuments,
    tributes to the Love we share.
There have been dark moments of my years,
Struggles against the shattered heart, scarred by the tears.

But now the Dreamer, the Searcher,
    the Wanderer in time
Loves and is Loved by the Golden Dancer
    — Eternity is mine.

For You,
Russ
November 1981
Cairo, Egypt

Obviously, there was little need for Russ and me to correspond with each other in the ensuing years of our marriage when we were never physically separated. But we did occasionally write each other love notes. Russ wrote one such note to me in 1992, early in our struggle to restore our marriage:

May 18, 1992
Dear Deb,
I've been thinking of sand dollars. Sometimes we didn't say much as we walked along the beach at Emerald Isle, but our hearts were talking. I loved those moments. The ocean winds blowing cold against us, demanding we pull each other closer. And, we did.

That beach — the walk, the wind, the sand — seems a lot like my life. Often the beach is torn by angry waves, the sand twisted with sad, ugly scars. A chill runs through me, driven by the tormented wind. It shoves me about, causing hurts and tears — trying to tear us apart.

But through it all, there is hope. I know what I'm looking for. I feel your warmth next to me, your eyes bright, your arm about me holding tight, and I smile.

There! I brush away the sand. We've found another sand dollar.

I Love You,
Russ

Ten

> Sometimes our light goes out but is blown into flame by another human being. Each of us owes deepest thanks to those who have rekindled this light.
>
> Albert Schweitzer

~~~~~~~~~~~~

Instruments Of Healing

In his essay, "Psychotherapists or the Clergy," the great Carl Jung wrote some 65 years ago, "Human thought cannot conceive any system or final truth that could give the patient what he needs in order to live: that is faith, hope, love and insight." He calls these "gifts of grace."[1] Sometimes gifts of grace come packaged in the form of loving friends or counselors who point us back to the light when we find ourselves wandering in the darkness.

Earlier, I offered a word of caution for those needing to select a counselor, regardless of background. I wish I could say that the post-modern age had been able to completely or even substantially close the gap between psychology and theology. In reality, the two are quite close, yet they appear so far apart. It's interesting to note that times haven't changed all that much since Jung wrote his essay and lamented this gulf himself. To him, the psyche was the spirit or the soul. He saw a great longing in people to fill the void created to some degree by 19th-century intellectual thought. The Freudian school, of which Jung was originally a part, but later castigated for its simple-mindedness, was in his words, "hostile to spiritual values."[2] Those therapists who disregarded man's spiritual side did then and still do today their patients a great disservice. Jung's words in the age between the two world wars still ring hauntingly true today: "It seems to me that, side by side with the decline of religious life, the neuroses grow noticeably more frequent. ... We are living undeniably in a period of the greatest restlessness, nervous tension, confusion and disorientation of outlook."[3]

I didn't have a Jung to counsel with, but I did have those who followed at least some of his line of reasoning. Psychology has come a long way as we hail the 21st century, but some things never change. I have made reference to several counselors of varying backgrounds who worked with me on my way to recovery from depression and various underlying issues. It may be helpful, or just plain enlightening, to know the progression of my therapy and to hear those therapists describe their own work. Perhaps this inside look at therapy can quell some of the fears and misgivings people have about it. There were four key people in the role of counselor or doctor. Each represented a different discipline. I engaged others along the way, but these four were the most helpful for me.

The first significant person to take an active role in my recovery process was my pastor, Rick Savage. My first real healing work was begun with him, and to an extent, with his wife, Vonnie. He has a real gift of empathy, but also the gift of perspective. In fact, I remember that word, PERSPECTIVE, appearing on a sign above his office door. Not only did he and Vonnie pray for and with me, but they enlisted the prayers of other believers. This umbrella of prayer was an essential part of my healing process. I could unashamedly call on Rick or Vonnie to stand with me during my trials when I knew my strength and my prayers alone were not sufficient. They were always there when I needed them. As a little child once said, we sometimes need God "with skin on."

Vonnie helped me to get through a situation that I might not otherwise have survived when my children were quite young and Russ was away on business once. She came to my house one evening when I was in the midst of a major depressive episode and helped me feed the children and put them to bed while seeing that I ate something, myself. She talked and prayed with me and helped me through my confusion, all this while she was still recovering from major surgery. Another couple, who were close friends, were similar angels of mercy on another occasion. I received a note from Vonnie after the trauma of my first major depressive episode in two years when our first daughter, Jennifer, was three months old:

> Dear Debbie,
> Just want you to know I love you and appreciate who you are! Your openness and honesty serve you well, and are a part of your healing process. I know that God is continuing His good work in you ... it is evident, even though you sometimes may not think so. Processes are sometimes slow and painful. Fun, no; a learning time, yes. Believe that God will turn it all around for your good as you continually commit yourself to serve Him.
> There is an acrostic I tell myself nearly every day:
>
> **D**aily
> **E**verything
> **L**aid
> **I**n
> **G**od's
> **H**ands
> **T**hankfully!
>
> Perhaps you've heard it before, but thought I'd share it again with you. You and Russ are super people, and we appreciate your friendship and support. Isn't it great to have each other in Christ's body? I continue to pray for you. Know I am here for you.
>
> Lovingly,
> Vonnie

I was so thankful to have Vonnie as a friend and Christian role model. Her loving affirmations contributed significantly to my recovery.

Pastor Rick used every means of communication at his disposal to encourage and help me, including notes, phone calls and personal visits. He sent me an article by Charles Allen entitled, "When You Get The Blues" during one of my worst bouts of depression along with a letter in which he detailed how he was praying for me. In essence, Allen wrote in that article about how we can lift ourselves out of depression by dwelling on ourselves as creations in the image of God and by remembering that we are needed to fulfill our unique roles in this world. We are to rise up, he reminds us, and "assert our authority" over the lesser entity inside that is vying for control of our best self. As a pilot in a spiraling aircraft, we are to pull up, not black out, by looking in hope toward God.[4] I was to recall that imagery many times when I wanted to bail out on myself and on God.

Hope was what I gained more of in my counseling with my pastor. Looking back on the times we spent together, Rick says he was giving me "emotional hugs." He told me as we reflected back on those days, "I remember thinking here was someone Vonnie and I really loved, but who was assuming responsibility for the blows that came your way. And you weren't responsible for the blows." He goes on to say today, "I remember thinking you were one of those persons who, every time while growing up you were ready to stand up straight, you'd get hit in the stomach. Before you could get your stature, you'd be hit again. Finally, it got easier to stay down because it hurt when you stood and exposed yourself. I thought you had come to a point in your life where you just didn't love yourself anymore. I wasn't a professional and I knew I couldn't take you the distance, but I began to think that somebody needed to love you unconditionally and try to convince you that not all of life is like that."

Pastor Rick knew how to be there for me, and even how not to be there:

> There were moments when you were really hurting. I think at those times we just looked at each other. We didn't really talk much because there wasn't much to do except to be together. And that's okay. You don't always need an instantaneous solution. I think true therapists will probably admit that they can't "fix it." We have to fix our own lives.

We can get guidance, input and help, but ultimately, we have to own our lives. Loneliness is perhaps the greatest enemy in the whole process. You do have to walk the journey alone. I wonder why some people bail out and you didn't. Perhaps because you realized that in your aloneness there were hands reaching out to you and people touching your life. Part of my job as a counselor and pastor is to know when to be there and when not to be. Some days, people just need to be alone. And then there are days when you need people around you.

He not only supported and loved me through my healing process, but he also provided emotional support for Russ. They had coffee together from time to time, and during those breaks, Russ would pour his heart out, affirming our relationship and receiving prayer and consolation from Rick. It was hard for him to know how best to be there for me. He needed counsel sometimes as much as I did.

Rick Savage has some other significant perspectives on my struggles. "Your experience was a confirmation of the grace of God for me," he says. "The days when you couldn't carry yourself, He carried you. When you wanted to throw in the towel, He was faithful. You had to walk through the nightmare — He didn't walk through it for you — but He didn't bail out on you. Your faith held you steady."

Pastor Rick and I both know that faith is the real pivotal point for emotional stability. I have had the privilege of praying for him and his family through some struggles of their own. "Faith enables you to pull back layers of hurt and deal with them one at a time," he observes. "Most of us mess up so badly by the time we get around to coming to God that for the rest of our lives we walk with a limp. God is always pulling back layers for us to look at and deal with so that we can get free." As I said earlier, the descent into the dark night of the soul and eventual re-emerging into the light is greatly liberating.

To paraphrase a great line from the movie, "The Natural," each of us has two lives: the life we learn with and the life we live with after we learn.[5] "I believe that," says Rick. "Today, I may feel on top of the world — healthy and mentally in shape — and God may be doing some great things in my life. But a week from today, something may happen that will cause me to realize another layer has just been exposed that I didn't know was there. I wasn't lying today. I thought I was okay. To me, that's not a sign of sin or weakness or vulnerability. It's actually a sign that I am in relationship with God. The closer I walk with Him, the more things in my life that aren't correct I'm going to see. I have to believe it was the grace of God in your life that brought you right up against the wall. In that moment, you may have wanted to say, 'God, I thought you loved me.' The real answer is, 'I do. That's why I've let you hit the wall. Now let's begin to work through things.'"

Chronologically, the next significant counselor to enter my life after my pastor was a lay counselor, Linda, who headed up a support group for women desiring to overcome depression, drug and alcohol addictions, eating disorders, child abuse and other emotional problems. We had all come from dysfunctional families, although our problems took different forms. Linda had, herself, recovered from severe depression. This made me feel particularly comfortable with her. Her emphasis was on the healing power of prayer and the Scriptures, while taking care of our physical needs. Her prescriptions encompassed the spiritual and the practical.

I spent just over a year in this group, and at the end of that time, I gave the experience mixed reviews. Linda did a masterful job of steering the group toward hope and healing. She used a sort of tough-love approach, telling us what we needed to hear and do. She used the Scriptures as her guide, and never pretended to be the ultimate authority. I sensed God's Holy Spirit in her, as well as her genuine love and concern for me. Proverbs tells us a friend's wounds are faithful. I know Linda was that friend. The negative feelings I experienced were directed at others in the group who I felt sometimes went off on tangents and sought to commiserate with each other more than find solutions to their problems. I sought to keep my journaling exercises concrete and relative to where I was at a given time, but some of my fellow group members succumbed to group pressure or some untenable need to dredge up pains or experiences they believed, rightly or wrongly, were buried deep in their subconscious memories in an effort to find release. It could create an atmosphere of surrealistic eeriness that I found alienating. I decided I would be better off in a one-on-one counseling situation. In truth, I also might have been a little afraid of being confronted in a group setting. My experience doesn't mean someone else wouldn't have a completely different perspective on this type of therapy. Each group must stand on its own merits. I believe that the benefit peaked for me after a year, which is probably as it should have been. I didn't need to be a support group junkie.

Group therapy is probably the most difficult type of treatment to assess in its effectiveness. While some groups seem to work rather well, admittedly, there are others that are ineffective and even unhealthy. I know of a church that found itself in the dubious position of having to monitor a recovery support group it sponsored when some unexpected negative feedback was received from some of those in attendance. Bickering and backbiting seemed the order of the day. My brother, Greg, during one of his more lucid moments recently told me he felt compelled to manufacture childhood problems under pressure from his peers in group therapy sessions. A person considering a support group of this type should go in with both eyes open. If you choose a group that turns out not to be what it appears, get out.

After my group experience, I began counseling with a psychologist whom I thought to be a Christian counselor. That's what she called herself. She had a delightful, magnetic personality, but I gradually came to see we had different spiritual reference points. Her philosophy veered too much toward the metaphysical for me. Here is another way in which needy patients can be duped if they are not wary. The best thing I can say about that arrangement was that through that person I was led to Dr. Bruce Hubbard, the psychiatrist who treated me for the biochemical disorder that no one else was clearly able to see. He is a good man, respected by his colleagues, and one who treated me from a purely medical perspective. I was not seeking spiritual counseling from him, though he affirmed my spirituality. There are excellent counselors and doctors who stand ready to help people battling depressive disorders, both biologically and emotionally. Sometimes a fear of being misled or misdiagnosed keeps people from seeking out those professionals, and I can understand that. I recommend being thorough and being willing to change courses if you're not satisfied with your treatment. That doesn't mean to bail out if you don't like doing the work. Healing doesn't come without some effort on your part.

The road to Dr. Hubbard was a long one, but the relief I felt was indescribable when he finally helped me to get on the right track. I mentioned earlier that another doctor had prescribed antidepressants for me about a year prior to my seeing Dr. Hubbard. He seemed to be treating them almost like aspirin. I felt I was being dismissed as a crazy, insignificant female by his "diagnosis." It was as if he were saying, "Take these and get yourself together, woman. I have more important patients to deal with." I dropped him from my list in a hurry. Not so with Dr. Hubbard. First, psychopharmacology was his specialty. Secondly, he was kind-hearted and took a genuine interest in me. He took into account my entire history. It was clear he took the Hippocratic oath — "First do no harm ..." — seriously. Our intermittent work together encompassed about five years and three phases. I still feel indebted to him.

Dr. Hubbard recalls our first meeting. "When I first saw you, it seemed to me that you were moderately depressed and slightly anxious. Although there were stresses in your life, with your children, with Russ and with your family, the degree of your symptoms was greater than you would expect of someone just facing those stresses. That's why I felt there was a biological component." Dr. Hubbard started me almost immediately on one common antidepressant, antianxiety medicine (amitryptiline or Elavil), which had limited success. He goes on to describe what happened next.

"About a year after that, it was clear that you were getting worse. That's when Russ came in with you. You were not functioning. You were withdrawing a lot during the day and you couldn't do anything. It was clear the medicine wasn't working." He recommended a second antidepressant, trazadone (Desyrel) — also commonly prescribed as a sleep aid and a pain killer — to which I had "almost a miraculous response."

It truly felt miraculous to me. This was the second phase of my treatment — finding the medicine that worked best with my chemistry for the symptoms of severe depression and anxiety. "Actually, you had as much anxiety as you did depression," recalls Dr. Hubbard. "You were fearful all the time and completely withdrawn." That is not an exaggeration.

The third phase of my therapy was working through the issues that came out after I became depression-free. Dr. Hubbard did some work with both Russ and me here, but he referred me to another therapist whom I worked with for several months (again, it wasn't the right mix) before I went on to Diane Eller-Boyko, whose work I briefly described in Chapter Eight.

During my years of counseling with Dr. Hubbard, I would drive about 40 miles to his office in San Diego. When I was only moderately depressed or not in a depressive episode, getting there was no problem. There were several occasions, however, when I was so impaired, I actually could not find my way to his office.

I mentioned earlier in this book that Dr. Hubbard considered me to be nonfunctionally, severely depressed at least 60 percent of the time. "That was a rough estimate," he says. "When you were at your worst, just before we put you on trazadone, I would say you were 99.9 percent depressed. In the month or two prior to changing your medicine, you were awful. I was really worried about you."

In those days, I was as close to being devoid of hope as a person can get and still live. To be honest, I didn't want to live. But my faith would not permit me to take my own life. I make an important distinction here between hope and faith. I have already said that it is difficult, if not impossible to feel hope during the depths of depression. The definition of despair is the lack of hope. But faith is an act of the will, not based on logic or evidence of things seen. A person can feel little or no hope, but still maintain faith in God, or even in other people. That faith will lead to action which will ultimately restore hope which will build even greater faith. That is a simple synopsis of my entire therapy and recovery.

Dr. Hubbard, to his credit, acknowledged my need to keep my therapy in a spiritual framework. Over the last 10 to 15 years, he maintains, psychiatry has recommended treating people in three spheres: the biological, the psychological and the social — the bio-psycho-social approach. "I think there's a fourth sphere," he adds, "and that's the spiritual. Finally, doctors are learning to recognize that. Rarely do we see a problem in one area that doesn't affect the other areas. All of these interact."

Dr. Hubbard is extremely optimistic in his outlook for his depressed patients, claiming, "I see that in 95 percent of the depressed people I treat, they recover and return to a normally functioning life. I see a lot of hope for them. It's hard to instill that in them when they're depressed because hopelessness is a major symptom of depression. When people try to re-establish their equilibrium emotionally, changes happen. When they're better, hope returns." Other therapists attest to slightly lower, but still highly impressive success rates. Dr. Hubbard seems to be a long-term therapist, which may account for the difference. Still, as Dr. James McCullough pointed out in Chapter Three, the permanent recovery percentages — what I call true healings — are not as high as those of people who are functionally recovered enough to return to their normal lives. Getting depressed people to recognize their problem and overcome their lack of trust in counselors can be challenging in some instances. I run into these people or their friends and family members all the time. When the trust relationship is established, healing can begin. For those people who have not yet acknowledged their spiritual underpinnings, these conditions may best exist initially in a non-religious environment. For those with traditional Judeo-Christian values, counseling that adheres to these principles will be more meaningful.

All reputable counselors should be nonjudgmental and compassionate, but they must hold you accountable to a standard of behavior. You're wasting your time and money if you meet with a counselor who allows you to establish your own moral code or who uses deceptive, feel-good tactics. I honestly don't know how many therapists prey on the vulnerabilities and the pocketbooks of their patients, but I know they exist. We all know the stories of people who have supposedly recovered repressed memories of early abuse under therapeutic hypnosis, only to find later that the "memories" were actually suggestions from their therapists. The same holds true of people whose diagnosed multiple personality disorder goes away when they quit or can no longer afford therapy.

My last phase of therapy, at the conclusion of which I stopped taking antidepressant medication, was largely accomplished with Diane Eller-Boyko, a licensed clinical social worker who is a Christian. I credit her with facilitating some major healing in me. Diane and I dealt a lot with all the defenses I had established since childhood to cover up my pain and disappointment. We looked at what is known as detaching from a parent because you perceive the parent can no longer meet certain ego-gratifying needs for one reason or another. In my case, this happened in some unique ways between my mother and me, though I also had the classic absentee father scenario to deal with. For those who have had any exposure to basic psychology at all, this discussion may sound a little Freudian. Remember that all modern psychology basically grew out of the schools of Freud, Adler or Jung. There are elements of validity to the ideas of all three, though Jung, to me, comes closest to getting it right. While he has been accused of drawing some of his beliefs from Gnosticism and occultism, many of his statements, taken at face value, are rational and have a good deal of validity to them, in my opinion.

I had always felt the lack of a relationship with my father was more at the root of my problems. While this was a major factor, the degree to which I felt I could be nurtured by my mother was also very significant to my emotional health. Diane believes when we experience this kind of detachment, "we pull into ourselves and therefore don't get our needs or egos gratified. When we come into our place of adulthood or even adolescence, we come into a need for independence, but that early need for nurturing is still there. We start to repress again and don't get needs met again and put up defenses."

Diane describes defenses as intellectualism, moralism and denial. "We say, 'This isn't me.' The thing is, it isn't, but we don't stop to think about what this is representing. We have some real needs that we're not going to look at because they're too threatening. So we push them away, and we move on. We're still living a life that is very repressed as far as a real sense of self or ego is concerned. It keeps rearing its head, but we're too frightened to look at it. The more we look at it, the more depressed we get. Our defenses keep us pretty locked up."

Diane and I reviewed my life's events until we got to my moment of crisis, which occurred in my first marriage. She goes on to say, "I think crises are a gift because they make our defenses have to shatter. It's a point where we take this opportunity of the will to say I'm going to move with this versus trying to resist this any longer. I'll let it take me wherever it needs to take me. It took you to doctors' offices, it took you to a chemical state that needed balancing out. Stress, repression or fear does something to our chemistry."

With Diane, I looked at my post-depression recovery period. As I felt better, I naturally socialized more and wanted to do more. In the process of opening up to my potential, I uncovered old, unmet needs. "These legitimate needs that you went through in development," explains Diane, " came into play and it was still pretty shaky because that part of you was not very well-formulated."

In my case, I had some very willful, rebellious responses to my nurturing needs. Even after I learned what they were all about, I wasn't immediately willing to let them go. This was the decision that brought the most pain to my marriage. I still don't fully understand it myself. But as Diane describes it, "You willingly let down those ego needs and said, 'a willingness, a surrender needs to take place here so that I can continue to grow and learn what God calls me to be.' I think your crisis was the anger, resentment and rebelliousness you were struggling with. The real crux of your therapy was working through this period of questioning and all those feelings of conflict. I can only imagine you had to say, 'No, I'm committed, I am not following this, I am surrendering, giving it up.' Then some real healing could start to happen. You were open to God, you were open to the graces in this world that He was offering you, that could become more gratifying than one can ever imagine."

When we seek a source outside ourselves that we perceive will bring us some kind of ego gratification, we're using what is known as an attachment. "It's a narcissistic search," says

Diane. "It can happen to anyone. We're all seeking, we're all hungering and thirsting for something to attach ourselves to, to give us a completeness, a oneness, a wholeness." These attachments, whatever they are, have a very powerful pull on us. They can be work for some, drugs or alcohol for others. In my case, it was a need for an emotional and physical bonding that, sad to say, I felt a need to seek outside of my marriage. The biggest hurdle that Russ and I both had to get over was understanding that this kind of attachment is not because of a physical need. Too many people make that mistake. There is always an emotional void in cases of marital infidelity. A healthy person has a good sense of self — the knowledge that they are separate from everyone else, not needing to merge with anyone else to become complete or know who they are. "I think an erotic experience is a way of calling us out to say, 'Who am I, what am I?'" summarizes Diane. "By bonding with this person in this way, somehow I get this union, this feeling of euphoria or well-being because when we mesh, we know who we are. It's a false sense of self. It was very destructive and would have been very destructive to your marriage, to your core, to your soul."

When we are in right relationship with God, I believe He will give us the true desires and needs of our hearts. My deep desire was to have a true friend, someone who would understand me and love and accept me unconditionally. I longed for a relationship with someone who was like me — a true kindred spirit. I believe this is a godly need, but for me it became an urgent one because I didn't grow up with real maternal intimacy. Bruno Bettelheim, recognized as one of the world's great child psychologists, addressed this need in women in an essay called "Growing Up Female" that originally appeared in *Harper's* in 1962: "The old intimacy between mothers and daughters who actually worked together for the survival of the family has now practically vanished. ... Many women now feel compelled to prove themselves good mothers by making sure their daughters are 'successes' in life, and so it is difficult for warm confidence to grow between them."

For a while, Russ was threatened by my need for this kind of feminine friendship. He felt that he should be my best friend and be able to meet my deepest emotional needs — and he does to the extent that any husband can do that. But women need other women as close friends. For years, I cried inwardly for this kind of friend. It wasn't until after I'd gotten back on my feet, so to speak, and was fairly healthy emotionally that this rare friend came into my life. She has been the most incredible blessing to me. It is more than mere coincidence that we were born only days apart or that she had a mentally ill mother and I a mentally ill father. We've both had some significant struggles in our lives. We both have two daughters very close in age who attended the same school. It was our children who brought us together. Until I met Janet, I'd been content to observe the special bond of sisterhood in my daughters, and I delighted in it. But now, I have a "sister" of my own and I understand the special love that God reserves for sisters. We have truly been therapeutic for each other and our bond is a lifelong one. Sadly, I had to leave her behind in California when I moved back to Virginia, but we've relied on cards, letters and occasional phone calls to keep in touch until we can see each other again.

It is rare to find friends who will provide a high degree of mutual accountability and unconditional love in today's postmodern world. I'm afraid I have to indict the church somewhat here, but I believe these kinds of relationships should be found in our churches, and of course in our families, first and foremost. That is not always the case. Too many churches are missing the boat when it comes to intervening in the lives of hurting people. There's little sense of community any more except for pockets here and there. We're so busy we jealously guard our privacy and respect others' private lives. How do we react when we learn that a beloved church member who was sitting in the pew in front of us last week went home and put a bullet in his head? Are we completely mystified, like the reader of E. A. Robinson's poem, "Richard Cory?" If only we'd known, we lament. Do we really know what we would have done? We should.

Russ and I have been blessed with a circle of faithful friends who believe in strengthening and preserving the family unit and each individual's worth, a cause to which I am deeply committed.

Rich DeVos, world-renowned business leader and cofounder of Amway Corporation, sums up the foundation of this philosophy in his first of 16 credos of compassionate capitalism:

> We believe that every man, woman and child is created in God's image, and because of that, each has worth, dignity and unique potential. Therefore, we can dream great dreams for ourselves and others.[6]

Who can argue with that? Following that statement with the simple postscript "... and we can love and affirm each other," gives us a recipe for whole and joyous living.

Eleven

Reading is the loom on which one's inner garments are woven.

A.P. Gouthey

~~~~~~~~~~~

Lessons From The Scribes

Norman Cousins has said, "Anyone who can read can learn how to read deeply and thus live more fully."[1] Cousins was known as somewhat of a renegade when he introduced literature into the courses he taught medical students at UCLA. He justified his decision thus: "Literature helps the medical student to analogize the patient, to make connections between the experiences of the race and the condition of the individual, and to fit the individual into a world that is less congenial than it ought to be for people who are more fragile than they ought to be."[2] Now some medical schools have taken the step of incorporating a spiritual element into the training of future doctors. I'm not sure what their definition of spiritual is, but it's a start.

There are many lessons to be gleaned from works of literature written by those who lived before us. Why shouldn't physicians know and utilize this? Mankind's struggles to understand this world and the fight against succumbing to despair in the face of life's frustrations make for some compelling themes in literature. Of course, these story plots are being lived out among us each day, sometimes in our very homes without our even knowing it.

I should make the point that I hold neither a psychiatry nor a psychology degree. But my English degree may be related when you consider the extent of critical analysis I was trained to perform on a plethora of literary works. Imagine the student of literature as Freud coaxing Franz Kafka onto the couch for a little psychoanalysis. Kafka, for you non-literary types, wrote, among others, a work called *The Metamorphosis*, which describes a man changed into a cockroach. When I was culling through college books, deciding which to keep for further edification, I threw Kafka out.

It has been said that the person you will become in five years is determined by the books you read and the people with whom you associate. There are those who think that statement might need a new millennium updating that replaces the phrase "books you read" with "movies and television programs you watch," or perhaps even "Internet sites you visit." While film and television may offer up some worthy fare, many scripts are simply rehashing classic literary themes or are based on books. A film simply cannot deliver as a book does, nor can it be studied in the same way. To listen to a certain major network's recent self-aggrandizing publicity spots is to be told condescendingly that television is the salvation of the world. The truth is something vastly different. Television executives know the world wide web is luring more and more people away from the tube — that is the ones who haven't already figured out better ways to spend their time. Still, we all hunger for a good story now and then and, whether we admit it or not, we really prefer to see it on the big screen in living color. Movies have always captivated us. They might be uplifting us, even helping to heal us more if we had more producers around today with Edgar J. Scherick's wisdom.

In 1996 when Russ and I edited a magazine we helped create called *ScreenWriter Quarterly,* Scherick contributed a commentary called "Write Yarns For Their Hungry Souls." Some of the sage advice he was giving to writers certainly bears repeating:

> Movie audiences are comprised of human beings and they are spiritually elevated when they see a member of their species acting with humanity. Humanity is our capacity for thought, memory and

feelings. It is what distinguishes us from every other animal species on earth. People in the name of humanity commit acts of bravery and compassion that are unique to our species. Other humans respond primordially to these acts of courage and compassion. ... Give the audience a reason to be proud of what they are. Help them to identify themselves with what is best in the species: courage and compassion, belief in what is right and proper as God gives us the ability to discern what is right and proper. ... And, when touched, the audiences will leave the theater anxious to share their experiences with others: the yearning, thrilling, healing — whatever it is that we bring to a boil within their hungry soul. ...[3]

Oh, for more Edgar Schericks! It's frustrating to note that in 1998 nearly two-thirds of the movies Hollywood produced were rated R or above while the average G-rated movie brought a 78 percent greater rate of return than the average R movie. Only six percent of movies made that year were rated G.[4] Is there a pattern here?

While the book market does have its share of meaningless fluff — some 60,000 new books are published every year — the greatest work of literature and the perennial best-seller remains the Holy Bible, which also happens to have inspired some great films. I read it as literature at sometimes stodgy Sweet Briar College, but having been raised just down the road in the Southern Bible Belt (I cut my teeth on Bible "sword drills" and was in church as a child two to three times a week), I was far more willing to accept Scriptural precepts at face value than my professors were. I'm not sure if my exposure to the liberal arts in college made it easier for me to veer off course later in life, but I did come to a point where I began to question some of what I had been spoon-fed as a child. Eventually, I came full circle and realized that truth was simpler than I had imagined. Perhaps it was my literary training that better equipped me to search out the truth for myself.

While the Old Testament, in particular, can be read as a

novel, I and many far wiser who have gone before me, don't believe for one moment that it is fiction. Believing the Bible as history would be a revelation to many people, who see this tome, in part, as just a collection of great, old, moral tales. Many other great works have drawn from the Bible's themes. It can be both comforting and scary to note that people have been dealing with the same universal struggles for many centuries. God, the creator's role in bringing order to the chaos of our lives is seen time and time again throughout biblical history. Great spiritual leaders of the Old Testament went through many trials during which their faith was tested. Who isn't familiar with the expression "the patience of Job?" The prophet Elijah, when fleeing from Queen Jezebel, experienced a dramatic shift from a victorious emotional high to the depths of despair so low that angels had to come and minister to him to save his life. Have you ever experienced this type of "rebound" depression? The lessons taught in these trials of old are the same lessons we are still learning today. Human beings have the same weaknesses, the same selfishness, the same fears as always. Wisdom has been called learning from the experiences of others. It seems we all have to acquire it the hard way, however.

Why did Thoreau write in 1854, "The mass of men lead lives of quiet desperation?"[5] Depression and despair aren't unique to modern society. We are more attuned to this age-old problem today, and unfortunately, much of the human race has lost its moral compass with the natural result being more hopelessness and despair. We have more reason to feel lost in this post-modern, stress-laden world. We have become more detached from others and from ourselves. Still, it's hard to imagine a more desperate plea than the psalmist, presumed to be King David, offered in Psalm 13. He was crying out to God, not to man:

> How long, O LORD?
> Will you forget me forever?
> How long will you hide your face from me?
> How long must I wrestle with my thoughts
> and every day have sorrow in my heart?
> How long will my enemy triumph over me?[6]

From Depression to Wholeness   175

I probably would have studied literature in college to the exclusion of all else, if my professors had allowed me to. I'm glad they didn't. I still have all my notebooks and papers from each course, as well as many of the books I read. Now, a quarter of a century later, I find them speaking to me again. They spent most of that time locked away in my attic, I have to admit. My professors would like me to say that I locked their precepts — at least the good ones — away in my consciousness. I'm sure some of them penetrated my gray matter.

Several English professors were influential in my impressionable life during my college years. One was a fellow by the name of Ross Dabney, now retired. He had an incredible penchant for memorizing and quoting long passages of poetry or prose. I remember him most, though, because he listened to me when I spoke to him of my past. He cared about who I was and where I was going. I confided to him that I wanted to write a book someday about my family struggles. This was a few years before the onset of my illness. He believed in me and encouraged me.

Another professor whom I respected, though whose somewhat liberal views I didn't always agree with, was Lee Piepho. His infamous advice when questioned about the length of an assigned paper was to "begin at the beginning and end at the end." I suppose that's a pretty good analogy of life. He was to have been my adviser in the junior honors program. He told me an honors project would probably provide the only meaningful knowledge I would retain from my college years. Sad, but true. I made excuses and dropped out of the honors program, however, before I really got started. This stands in my mind today as one of my first great failures. I think I punished myself by taking an advanced Latin course the following year. I never worked harder in my life! (I retained very little of it, by the way, but I do remember being humiliated by an upper classman when I mispronounced "Descartes" in a religion class discussion. I blame it on all that Latin). Even though Professor Piepho saw in me the potential to excel, I couldn't see it in myself. I simply could not see myself as a college honors student. I've had a difficult time forgiving myself for quitting all these years. That shame became a turning point in my life, and was one of the driving factors behind my will to succeed and make a name for myself in the Marine Corps.

I could never forget the late Ralph Aiken, who set a high — and sometimes frustrating — standard for me and urged me on to do my best, even when I felt as if I were drowning in a sea of obscure literature. I was among those who received what must have been his highest compliment on a critical paper — "This is sensible to searching ... and even well-written" — though, to be sure, I was not his best student. As scholarly as he was, he did not belittle my desire to pursue a career of journalism, a gesture for which I am still grateful. Known as a master stylist and one thoroughly familiar with his subject matter, Dr. Aiken's arcane airs could be unsettling. I must confess that they endeared him to me however. He endowed me with a deep appreciation of English — which he distinctly separated from American — literature. I don't think he wanted us to know that England had given rise to both tories and whigs. Otherwise, he had plenty to say about the Brits. The only time I ever saw the man near speechless was when I announced to him that I was going to become a Marine officer.

I had earlier mentors who are to be commended for their influence on my life. Three of these individuals are still living. Two were teachers — Erma Burch and Eva Hartless, my fourth and sixth grade mentors, who loved their calling — and one was my elementary school principal for several years, Nathaniel "Nick" Habel. My little country school was rather unique. While Christian influences were being removed systematically from American public schools and the Cold War was being waged (an irony if ever there were one), our hearts were still being molded through the time-honored values that were an extension of our close-knit, rural community. Mr. Habel was a man who personified joy and true praise to me — a real Psalm 66 kind of guy. He led us in song, even hymns, during our weekly chapels — we didn't call them assemblies. I had the privilege of hearing him as a guest preacher recently, the first time I'd seen him in 35 years. He chose one of my favorite New Testament chapters, Philippians 4, the letter through which Paul expounds on joy, inner strength and harmony within the church. He resurrected a familiar truism about attitudes that has circulated for years: "Some people are born in the objective case and live in the subjunctive mood." Any good student of English grammar can appreciate that. We all know those weaned-on-a pickle-face people. Though we don't always recognize it, sometimes they look back at us from the mirror.

It was my mom, who was an English teacher, but perhaps even more my aunt, her teacher-sister, who fed my love of literature when I was a child. Some of the more pleasant memories I have as a child are of the times I spent curled up with a good book, on some armchair adventure or another. Books were my solace and escape from the pressures of an unhappy family life. I read everything from classics to biographies to historical fiction. I particularly liked mysteries. Many of the innate truths I carry with me today came from my early reading, which also included Bible stories. I still remember exactly where I was and the book I was reading — *Old Yeller* — the moment I received the painful news that my beloved Aunt Edith had died a premature death from a heart attack. That book was a perfect one to console myself with at the age of 11.

There are numerous, much-loved youthful heroes and heroines portrayed in children's literature. While my adolescent daughters sometimes get stuck in a rut of *Nancy Drew* or *Thoroughbred* stories, I encourage them to read children's classics. I have to fight their inclinations to watch the movie versions, however. One of my favorite stories is *The Secret Garden* (both the book and film versions) with its indomitable, young protagonist, Mary Lennox. Orphaned at 10 and sent to live with her reclusive and often-absent uncle, she encounters Colin, the cousin she never knew she had. Their mothers were twin sisters, each having died an untimely death. Sickly since his premature birth, Colin is sequestered in a dark, hidden room, pale and believing himself unable to walk or ever leave his bed. He is constantly pampered and ministered to by the household servants, who have convinced him he will die young. Mary sees him as a spoiled, fearful child and refuses to put up with his nonsense. When Colin announces to Mary, "I am going to die," she replies, "How do you know?" He tells her, "Oh, I've heard it ever since I can remember. ... They are always whispering about it and thinking I don't notice. They wish I would, too." "If they wished I would," Mary retorts, "I wouldn't."[7] Through her eyes, her cousin comes to see himself and the world as alive and full of wonder. The secret garden that Mary discovers and brings back to life becomes a metaphor for Colin's renewal and his restored relationship with his father. It's a story with lessons for young and old, alike.

I particularly like didactic, even allegorical literature and we all enjoy diversion and entertainment. A good writer can take us into an enchanted world and show us something about ourselves without making us aware he's done it. We may see something of our baser side or discover truths that elevate humanity and us as individuals. Reading an uplifting book or story can help anyone who is mired in depression or prone to get that way. Likewise, reading the wrong kinds of books — tragic, unredemptive stories or tales of horror— can make us more anxious or depressed. I highly recommend that parents monitor the kinds of things your children are reading, watching and listening to. If you're allowing them to play violent video games or listen to Marilyn Manson and those of his ilk, you're making a tragic mistake. There is no compromise here. Period. We suffer as a society today because we no longer read for universal knowledge and personal edification. We want to be coddled and entertained. Or we want to taste the fruit of the forbidden tree — to live as close to the edge as we can.

We need to be as concerned about our emotional and spiritual well-being as we are about our physical health. Public pressure has forced the cigarette industry to place warnings on its packaging. Alcoholic beverages and establishments that serve them must at least alert expectant mothers to the danger alcohol poses to their unborn children. The Food and Drug Administration places ingredient listings on food packaging so that those who must watch their diets for health reasons will be informed. Where are the warnings for music, video, books, magazines and all the trashy offerings any of us can consume at will? "Warning! Exposure to this product can cause addiction, despair, violence, impaired relationships and death to the soul." The health gurus want us to live forever, but to what end? Do they ever tell us what we're living for?

Thankfully, I was given some clues when I was young so that I might answer that question eventually. My love of reading made it only natural that I would pursue an English degree in college. My favorite place to hang out on campus was the library. I not only spent many hours studying there, but I also was employed part-time as a library assistant. Somehow, I felt safe down in the stacks among countless shelves of books. I felt warm and secure in the Browsing Room, with its rich, paneled walls, especially on a rainy day. Books were my friends. I've never felt more stimulated than when doing research, a trait I've since learned is attributable to my largely melancholy temperament. I felt rewarded somehow when I was able to obtain that old copy of Burton's *Anatomy of Melancholy* just by being in the right place at the right time.

Why would I be so drawn to a centuries-old book on the study of depression? If I knew the answer to that question, I would also know why I took a course called "Literature of Disillusionment" in the dreary January winter term. It could have been because I liked being in Ross Dabney's class or because we got to sit around on sofas and fluffy pillows and drink Chinese tea during class, so we would be less depressed, I suppose. We read such works as Kafka's *The Metamorphosis* or Conrad's *Heart of Darkness*. I actually enjoyed the class, and got an A in the course. Scary.

Many authors and artists share the melancholy temperament trait, not to be confused with melancholia or the state of being depressed, although plenty of artisans have suffered from that, too. There is a prevailing myth that the greatest artists have manic-depressive tendencies and that they are at the height of their creativity in states of mania. Kathy Cronkite quotes Dr. John Kelsoe in her book, *On the Edge of Darkness*, as saying, "If you eliminated bipolar genes from the population, who knows what other beneficial effects you might be losing, even beyond creativity?"[8] That observation is not without some truth. Nevertheless, I can illustrate its antithesis. Russ and I have a highly creative and successful screenwriter friend who makes himself adhere to a strict, sometimes monotonous schedule of writing. He doesn't smoke or drink and keeps very little on which to binge in his refrigerator. He is as even-keeled as they come and debunks the myth of chaotic creativity. It just doesn't have to be that way.

To better understand the temperaments that govern us all, I recommend reading Tim LaHaye's books, *Understanding the Male Temperament* (women, it can help you, too — it's mostly generic) and *Why You Act the Way You Do*. There is a down side to the melancholy temperament which can override its strength. While people like me are generally highly sensitive to the pain and joy of others and emote this empathy in their relationships, they tend to get down on themselves and others, too. You don't have to look far to find disillusioned philosophies of life in the works that melancholy artists produce. To the extent that art mirrors life, they may reflect the depression-prone people of our society.

Vincent van Gogh was an interesting case study. He clearly had a melancholy temperament and suffered from depression so great he was confined to an asylum for a period near the end of his life. In fact, his acclaimed work, "The Starry Night" (the one mentioned in the lyrics of Don McClean's 1971 song), was painted from his asylum room as he looked through his barred window, about a year before he committed suicide, eventually becoming immortalized in that bizarre way that Marilyn Monroe or Elvis Presley did. His story is as responsible as any for giving rise to the myth of the deranged artist. We can see van Gogh as both a painter and a writer through the 690 yellowed letters he wrote to his younger brother, Theo. He writes of himself, "My head is sometimes heavy, and often it burns and my thoughts are confused. ... My stomach has become terribly weak."[9] Does that not sound a lot like the words written by the writers of the Psalms to describe their pain? Oddly enough, van Gogh once sought to pursue seminary studies. He also wrote to Theo once, "There is a God Who knows what we want better than we do ourselves, and Who helps us whenever we are in need."[10] Many deep thinkers contemplate God and His purpose for life in a profound and philosophical way, while sadly never really knowing Him.

A clear genius, van Gogh lived a life not unlike that of my younger brother. A *National Geographic* expose´ quotes Dr. Peter Hanneman, director of the Psychiatric Crisis Center in

Amsterdam, the city which houses the Van Gogh Museum, as saying, "Most helpful for such a person would be to help him find that part of himself he does not ordinarily use. ... If he finds it, his so-called problems can disappear or seem less important."[11] Would that unused part be a person's spiritual identity? There is a poignant and ironic truth to a statement written in one of Vincent's letters. I've seen it quoted in various places. It's one of those little golden apples, almost suitable for embroidering on a sampler: "The best way to know God is to love many things."[12] It's true we can know God through His creation, but we can also know ourselves by choosing to love ourselves. After all, we are His greatest creation.

I have adopted a much more optimistic outlook on life than I used to have, thankfully, having worked to strengthen the sanguine or more outgoing part of my temperament. However, I found that in the academic world, a person with a melancholy temperament could have his or her disillusionment fed without having to go very far. Actually, I started out in my early days of formal education as more of a sanguine child, but a year or two of public schooling changed that. It only took one or two occasions of being ridiculed in front of my peers by an ignorant and insensitive teacher to frighten the spontaneity right out of me. My self-image was largely shaped by those unfortunate early learning experiences.

By the time I got to college, my self-image hadn't improved much. I still could be easily intimidated, but I began to blossom more as I approached my senior year. I chose to compare and contrast two works that on the surface seem to be very disparate for my senior comprehensive evaluation in English. One was Eugene O'Neill's modern play, *Long Day's Journey into Night*; the other was Jane Austen's 19th-century novel, *Persuasion*. This examination was supposed to evaluate our knowledge of and sensitivity to a wide spectrum of art forms and literary devices and our ability to write critical analyses (psychoanalyses?).

O'Neill's "play of old sorrows," as he called it, is a classic example of family psychodrama based on his own unhappy younger life. The story centers around a New York Irish Catholic family trying to cope with a wife and mother who is a drug addict. The younger of the adult sons (O'Neill) has tuberculosis. The entire family drown their sorrows in alcohol and continually criticize one another while trying to figure out how to love one another. One doesn't find much of redemptive value in the play, unless it's in the form of contrasting who we should be with who the characters are. I suppose I was drawn to it because of my own family situation. As O'Neill eventually forgave his family the pain they caused him, I have learned to forgive mine. The characters in his play are pathetically tragic. Mary, the drug addict, sums up her disillusioned view of life:

> None of us can help the things life has done to us. They're done before you can realize it, and once they're done, they make you do other things until at last everything comes between you and what you'd like to be, and you've lost your true self forever.[13]

There are a lot of Marys walking around in the world today.

Edmund, the unhealthy son, is likewise tormented by the family's shared pain when he laments about his mother's unlikely recovery: "They never come back! Everything is in the bag! It's all a frame-up! We're all fall guys and suckers and we can't beat the game!"[14]

Mary despairs of life as she reflects on her hopeless situation:

> I never lied about anything once upon a time. Now I have to lie, especially to myself. But how can you understand when I don't myself? I've never understood anything about it, except one day long ago I found I could no longer call my soul my own.[15]

Those lines express the anguish and the capitulation of the depressed mind. I don't think I could verbalize it any better if I tried. I particularly saw my one-time need to lie to and about myself in Mary.

Much more endearing, because they were written with a different purpose, are Jane Austen's novels with their admirable heroines. They are women of character who face disappointments, but strive to rise above them with dignity. Her stories are heroic and dignified. In fact they've enjoyed a latter-day revival, particularly in motion picture versions, one script even winning an academy award for its screen adapter. I always felt elevated for having read Austen's books.

By far, her best-loved and most worthy heroine is Anne Elliot in *Persuasion*. Anne is 28 and single, her plans to marry her true love having been thwarted by the lady who became her adviser after the death of her mother. The former object of her affections, now a naval captain, returns after eight years, secretly hoping to resume his suit. They discover each has remained faithful to the other and eventually realize that they can never again be parted by social convention. It's a simple story, but one driven by the sea of complex, private emotions that Anne must navigate as she strives to live a life of propriety and steadfast character in order to win back the man who seems her perfect match. I realized many years later how reminiscent my own journey to be with the Marine officer I loved was of Anne's plight — though I could only aspire to her lofty character at the time. The climactic letter that Captain Wentworth writes to Anne, finally revealing his true feelings for her, has more than a little of the flavor of Russ' written declaration of love to me, composed on a naval vessel sailing from England to Norway.

There is a good-natured debate near the end of the novel on the depth and longevity of love from both a feminine and masculine perspective between Anne and Captain Harville, who is a respected and honorable protagonist. It is all the more interesting because it takes place while Captain Wentworth, in the same room, is surreptitiously (also unknown to the reader) writing the aforementioned love letter that Anne will soon read. Through Anne, Austen offers an insightful look into why women — or at least those in a more traditional role — may become depressed more often than men:

> We certainly do not forget you so soon as you forget us. It is, perhaps, our fate rather than our merit. We cannot help ourselves. We live at home, quiet, confined, and our feelings prey upon us. You are forced on exertion. You have always a profes-

sion, pursuits, business of some sort or other, to take you back into the world immediately, and continued occupation and change soon weaken impressions.[16]

Austen's novels portray a world which reflects her distaste for shallowness and hypocrisy. She penned characters who embody the weaknesses of human nature as foils for those who speak for honor, integrity and marital bliss. Her world — rural England and its gentry, unblighted as yet by industrialism — stands in great contrast to the society that, say, Charles Dickens would later describe. Being a country girl at heart, and one of mostly English/Scottish extraction, I am easily drawn into Austen's novels. She writes of hope and redemption and of a resilient human spirit, so unlike the disillusioned and tormented souls seen in *Long Day's Journey into Night* or many of the nihilistic works of modern playwrights or novelists. One writer I know of claims she first became depressed as an adolescent when she read the works of Camus and Sartre. No adolescent should even know these works exist!

Austen's novel and O'Neill's play are merely two works of literature among a vast sea of works that represent either the hope or the despair of society. I cite them here because of the unique place they hold in my history. *Persuasion* I can take great delight in rereading many times. *Long Day's Journey into Night* I would read again only if I had to. The obvious lesson I retain from both these works is that it is far better to take ownership of your life and have hope than to acquiesce to despair or apathy.

I read many authors while in college and gained an appreciation for all the knowledge stored in those books. I read Horace and Juvenal in Latin, a language now all but lost to the modern world, yet once spoken by a culture which contributed greatly to many of the world's other languages. I was intrigued by references to the early church and to the first Christians in the very words that were written in that day. I read the theologies and philosophies of St. Augustine, Locke and Kierkegaard — and, yes, Descartes (pronounced Day-CART). I worked my way through Chaucer, Milton, Shakespeare, early and modern poets (learning to my delight that one of my alleged 17th-century English ancestors was a main subject in a famous political satire of Dryden's), early and modern novels and early and modern drama. I even became a fan of Samuel Johnson, the famed 18th-century English scholar, sage, poet and author who was unashamed to profess his Christian faith, unorthodox as it might have been at times. Dr. Johnson, as he is more often called, suffered the affliction of depression for much of his life. He managed to remain creative through some of his depressive episodes, a fact I find amazing (again, debunking the mania myth). But he was too disciplined to let his mind lie unused and open to depressive thinking, believing that work and good company were his only way of coping, a mode of thinking totally foreign to a post-modern, feelings-oriented society. I recently reread major portions of James Boswell's famous *Life of Johnson*, and was even more taken with it than when I originally read it in college. I admit, not everybody can appreciate 18th-century history or thought, and it probably constitutes a foreign language to most Bridgers and Generation Xers. I dare say if more of us endeavored to study it — and the birth of the American nation, which was an 18th-century event of great magnitude — we would be the better for it.

Dr. Johnson gave the world some magnificent gifts in the form of the written word. Even his letters and prayers are a delight to read. I can't help indulging in a Johnsonian sampler:

> Wherever human nature is to be found, there is mix of vice and virtue, a contest of passion and reason; and ... the Creator doth not appear partial in his distributions, but has balanced, in most countries, their particular inconveniences by particular favours.

> Friendship, peculiar boon of heav'n,
> The noble mind's delight and pride,
> To men and angels only giv'n,
> To all the lower world deny'd.

> A man who writes a book, thinks himself wiser or wittier than the rest of mankind; he supposes that he can instruct or amuse them, and the publick

to whom he appeals, must, after all, be the judges of his pretensions.

It is a sad reflection, but a true one, that I knew almost as much at eighteen as I do now. My judgement, to be sure, was not so good; but I had all the facts.

And, my favorite:

(A note following a prayer entitled *On the Study of Philosophy, as an Instrument of Living*): This study was not pursued.[17]

Is there any wonder why I still love the delightful and controversial Dr. Johnson? He was a fighter and a survivor, and a man of deep conviction. To be sure, I would have been held in great contempt for my past sins by this outspoken gentleman. He viewed a woman as more culpable in crimes of domestic moral turpitude. In his day, women were viewed as subject to their husbands under the strict interpretation of Ephesians 5:22. "Confusion of progeny constitutes the essence of the crime," said Johnson, with characteristic circular reasoning.[18] It's amusing to note that I am reputed to be the illegitimate progeny of Anthony Ashley Cooper, the First Earl of Shaftesbury, a nobleman who was born about a century before Dr. Johnson, and certainly one he would have known about. Shaftesbury's indiscretions were not lost to history, but somehow my apparent ancestors managed to keep the bloodlines straight. After all, it was blue blood.

A writer most highly respected by the intellectuals of academia and by Christians, alike, and one well-acquainted with the works of Dr. Johnson, is the late C. S. Lewis. He has been called "the ideal persuader for the half-convinced, for the good man who would like to be a Christian but finds his intellect getting in the way."[19] Medieval and Renaissance literature are among my favorite genres, and it was through his literary commentaries that I came to know Oxford and Cambridge Universities' Professor Lewis. An Anglican in his youth, but later an atheist, he was a man of reason who became a Christian by first setting out to disprove Christianity. He is probably best known to younger readers for his allegorical *Chronicles of Narnia.* His nonfiction writings are, themselves, works of art. In his book, *Mere Christianity,* Lewis has some things to say about human weakness and the tendency to acquiesce to life's struggles:

> One must train the habit of faith. The first step is to recognise the fact that your moods change. The next is to make sure that, if you have once accepted Christianity, then some of its main doctrines shall be deliberately held before your mind for some time every day. That is why daily prayers and religious reading and church going are necessary parts of the Christian life. We have to be continually reminded of what we believe. Neither this belief nor any other will automatically remain alive in the mind. It must be fed.[20]

If good thoughts must be fed continually to "remain alive" in our minds, does it not also follow that negative, self-destructive thoughts must likewise be fed to maintain a hold on us? Depressed people have a tendency to continually feed this negative side of themselves to keep it alive. As C. S. Lewis says, we can abate some of this undesirable despair by simply changing our habits. Reading, and particularly, biblical reading can help us accomplish this.

Thoreau, in an essay published posthumously in 1863 — "Life Without Principle" — hit the nail squarely on the head when he wrote about profane thoughts and shallow influences (one of which he considered to be, as I do, daily newspapers):

> By all kinds of traps and sign-boards, threatening the extreme penalty of the divine law, exclude such trespassers from the only ground which can be sacred to you. It is so hard to forget what it is worse than useless to remember! If I am to be a thoroughfare, I prefer that it be of the mountain-brooks, the Parnassian streams, and not the town sewers. There is inspiration, that gossip that comes to the ear of the

attentive mind from the courts of heaven. ... Knowledge does not come to us in details, but in flashes of light from heaven. Yes, every thought that passes through the mind helps to wear and tear it, and to deepen the ruts.

Little did Thoreau know how accurately he was describing the brain's neurobiological reaction to negative input. He was just exercising common sense, much of which has fallen by the wayside today.

Biblical reading takes on a wholly new dimension for one who has prayerfully sought God's wisdom and understanding of the Scriptures. In the Bible, we can both have our humanness affirmed and be inspired to rise above human frailty. Going back to the Psalms, which Martin Luther called a "little Bible," we see a collection of "the deepest and noblest utterances" of the saints to God. A full range of emotions is expressed by the Psalmists. In his *Preface to the Psalms*, Luther says:

> The human heart is like a ship on a stormy sea driven about by winds blowing from all four corners of heaven. In one man, there is fear and anxiety about impending disaster; another groans and moans of all the surrounding evil. One man mingles hope and presumption out of the good fortune to which he is looking forward; and another is puffed up with a confidence and pleasure of his present possessions. Such storms, however, teach us to speak sincerely and frankly, and make a clean breast.

Luther would certainly have had great interest in the Psalms' consolation considering he struggled with depression in his own life. We can take much comfort, and I have, in reliving both the pain and the joy contained in the Psalms. The psalmists, we are reminded by Rabbi Harold Kushner in his book, *Who Needs God*, had the "ability to find God in the sun and in the storm."[21] It feels okay to be a frail human, often ruled by emotions, when reading King David's and other psalmists' supplications to God in their hours of greatest need. The Psalms of praise lift our spirits and help us remember what awesome creations we are and how much God loves us. Again, I defer to Martin Luther:

> When the Psalms speak of fear or hope, they depict fear and hope more vividly than any painter could do, and with more eloquence than that possessed by Cicero or the greatest of the orators. And, as I have said, the best of all is that these words are used by the saints in addressing God; that they speak with God in a tone that doubles the force and earnestness of the words themselves. For when a man speaks to another man on subjects such as these, he does not speak from his deepest heart; his words neither burn nor throb nor press as urgently as they do here.

To whom else can we turn to "speak from [our] deepest heart"? The tri-partite Godhead, comprising the Father, Son and Holy Spirit, is our best counselor. Of course, it can take a while to learn to listen, but we are told He hears us even when we cannot form coherent thoughts, and "intercedes for us with groans that words cannot express."[22] When we can only communicate unspeakable pain to God, He understands. There is no friend so gifted.

Of all the books in the world, I firmly believe we should take the time to acquaint or reacquaint ourselves with the Bible, in fact, to study it. All the truth we may ever need to know is in this one volume. A century or two ago, it was unthinkable for any person of reason not to be familiar with biblical truths. Thomas Jefferson, though he could never accept the validity of anything miraculous and pasted together his own version of the New Testament, understood the importance of Jesus' teachings. He incorporated those "self-evident" truths into the Declaration of Independence and other writings. Especially within the last 30 years or so, those truths have been stripped of their self-evidence. If scientists, many of whom are agnostics or atheists, can still acknowledge the Bible to be inerrant in its conformity to the laws of physics and astronomy, perhaps we laymen can accept that its spiritual teachings just might also validate modern psychology.

I am fascinated by a verse in the book of Hebrews, which in the Greek translation, takes on a significant meaning with psychological implications. Hebrews 4:12 says "For the word of God is living and active. Sharper than any double-edged sword, it penetrates even to dividing soul and spirit, joints and marrow; it judges the thoughts and attitudes of the heart." The Greek word that is translated as "active" here is *energes* meaning engaged in work or effective. It is actually a medical term. The word of God as revealed in the Scriptures, the "double-edged sword," then is more of a surgeon's scalpel which penetrates all the way to the heart, cutting away harmful, cancerous thoughts and attitudes which can make our bodies and souls sick — and even kill us. There is no more potent example of the power of the Word than this.

If one looks around and observes the glories of nature and the laws of science, it is difficult to believe that the world, and those who people it, were not created by design. The more we observe, the more we have to be convinced. It is interesting to note the tenets of scientific creationism, as put forth by the scientists who established the Institute of Creation Research. One of them states, "Although people are finite, and scientific data concerning origins are always circumstantial and incomplete, the human mind (if open to the possibility of creation) is able to explore the manifestations of that Creator rationally and scientifically, and to reach an intelligent decision regarding one's place in the Creator's plan."[23]

Today, 40 percent of American scientists profess their belief in a personal God.[24] Science and theology are seen as more compatible than ever before. Nature cries out, telling us there must be a God and that He is awesome and powerful. "When you realize that the laws of nature must be incredibly finely tuned to produce the universe we see, that conspires to plant the idea that the universe did not just happen, but that there must be a purpose behind it," says John Polkinghome, former Cambridge physicist turned Anglican priest.[25] Psalm 19 reminds us of this truth: "The heavens declare the glory of God" (the Hebrew word is El, the generic name for God, the Creator).[26] But nature can't tell us what God wants or how we are to relate to Him. That's why we need His Word, life's Big Book of Instruction. Later in Psalm 19, we read "the law of the LORD is perfect, reviving the soul; The precepts of the LORD are right, giving joy to the heart. ... By them is your servant warned; in keeping them there is great reward."[27] The reference to God as LORD (all capitalized) means Yahweh (Yhwh) or Jehovah, the covenant God of Israel. This is the God with whom we have relationship, even today.

There is much comfort in the Psalms, and in many of the healing and instructive words of Jesus Christ in the New Testament, for the depressed person. If all else has failed you, this might be a good place to direct your attention. I encourage you to pray for wisdom to understand the Scriptures rather than approaching them with trepidation. This Divine enlightenment is one of God's mysteries. Remember, "He has given us His very great and precious promises, so that through them you may participate in the divine nature and escape the corruption in the world caused by evil desires."[28]

I think the book of Psalms is a great place to stay focused if you're just beginning to read the Bible. There are psalms that teach about Israel's history, that celebrate creation and the works of God. Many are testaments to His power and righteousness. God's compassion and faithfulness to His people also can be grasped through the psalmists. The Psalms are quoted significantly in the New Testament. As the Apostle Paul says in Romans, "For everything that was written in the past was written to teach us, so that through endurance and the encouragement of the Scriptures we might have hope."[29]

I also would point readers toward 1 John in the New Testament, an intimate look at the believer's relationship with God, the father written by the Apostle John. We are spoken of in this tender book as "little children," the Greek term being *teknia*, meaning *born-ones*. It has been said that John's Gospel leads across the threshold of the Father's house, but his First Epistle makes us at home there.

When we want to dwell on painful memories that tend to separate us from God's wholesome purpose for us, we can reconnect by reading the Bible and focusing again on the great God of history. When He seems temporarily absent in our lives, we need only tell ourselves, "I will remember the deeds of the LORD; yes, I will remember your miracles of long ago."[30] God is still working miracles all around us every day — yes, the same God who brought the rebellious children of Israel out of Egypt and into the Promised Land. If God is leading you through a desert, like He led the Israelites, just remember He *is* leading. Perhaps it is a desert of your own choosing; perhaps it is not. He has had a purpose for you, just as He did His children back then — "to humble you and to test you in order to know what was in your heart, whether or not you would keep His commands."[31] It is not God's desire to see His children denied their birthright. He offers us the key, but we must take it. When all is said and done, God's rules are still the best rules, leading us to that otherwise elusive peace "which surpasses all comprehension. ..."[32]

Epilogue

From Psalm 119

I know, O LORD, that Thy
judgments are righteous,
And that in faithfulness Thou
hast afflicted me. (v. 75)
It is good for me that I was afflicted,
That I may learn Thy statutes. (v. 71)
If Thy law had not been my delight,
Then I would have perished in my affliction.
I will never forget Thy precepts,
For by them Thou hast revived me. (vv. 92-93)[1]

In my garden is a small rose bush that I started from bare root. It is a reminder of God's order and dominion. I see myself in it. The roots took hold and grew slowly at first, even under less-than-ideal conditions. The plant looked all but dead for months. I was tempted to yank it out of the life-giving ground for lack of patience. But one day, after checking just one more time, I saw the first tiny shoots finally appear. Healing is like that. It still amazes me when any tender shoot pushes its way through the hard, spring ground. Like those plants, we are all stronger than we appear.

If you are seeking a healing from a depressive disorder, you have a journey ahead of you. Just how many steps you will have to take I can't say. You've heard it said that a journey of a thousand miles begins with the first step. This book may only be a catalyst to your admission of humanness. Just remember this is a journey that you don't have to take alone. While, as Pastor Rick Savage reminded me, we all own our lives and ultimately make our own choices, there are people who love you and will walk with you on the road to recovery. They are waiting to be asked for their help. Ask them ... and ask God. He owns our souls.

My main mission in writing this book, along with demystifying depression, has been to show people how to keep despair from seeping into their hearts and souls and robbing them of the God-given joy that is their birthright. That doesn't mean that we are to deny the pain and sorrow that comes into every life from time to time. We just don't memorialize it.

There is no one simple formula, no magic pill that works for everyone. But I believe with all my heart there is a solution for everyone. God knows every heart and its unique needs. If the answer lies mainly in any one of the four spheres I (and my counselors) have talked about — the biological, the psychological, the social or the spiritual — by now you must know that I believe it is the spiritual, from which all the others emanate. Public awareness — and science — have tended to revolve more around the other three, however. One sphere is predominantly influencing the others in most cases of depression, but in order to experience wholeness, it is helpful to be aware of and deal with all of them.

As I have attempted to make clear, science and theology are compatible — actually dependent upon each other. Science can only explain part of what God created. God would hardly be God if we could fully understand Him. Because man's spiritual sphere is so little understood, it is often shortchanged. While these divine concepts may be harder for some to digest, they can't just be dismissed. A person who has experienced a healing of any kind begins to feel more connected with the spiritual side of his or her being. If you become that person, down the road, you may find yourself looking back and understanding some of the signposts that you couldn't see or comprehend as you walked by them. In so doing, you will gain a new level of maturity that will enable you to reach out and help others you may encounter, extending the hand of "recycling grace."

Consider this observation made by Hugh Prather in his *Notes on Love and Courage:*

> We are born into a life. The life is waiting there. We don't pick it, we step into it: parents, first born or last, the part of the country, the part of the world, our

appearance, the efficiency of our brain. Then a time comes when we realize that we also have choices, and so we start the task of building our own life — an impossible task considering the number of days we are given to complete it. However, I don't think that's important; what is important is to begin.[2]

Just as we can't lay the cornerstone in building our lives, we don't get to add the finishing touches, either. That's the Master Builder's job, and He does it perfectly. "He who began a good work in you will carry it on to completion until the day of Christ Jesus."[3] This assurance will keep you on your journey.

Appendix

Ten Tips for Conquering Depression

Advice for the Depressed Person:

1. Don't try to ignore your symptoms of excessive sadness, anxiety or low energy. They could point to either a serious physical illness or clinical depression. Tell a doctor. Analyze the stress factors in your life. You may be on overload.

2. If you are depressed, resist the desire to isolate yourself from others. Confide your feelings to your spouse, a close friend or other caring family member.

3. Take a walk and commune with God and nature or participate in some other physical activity. Moderate exercise relaxes muscles and stimulates the release of endorphins, the body's natural antidepressants, and other mood enhancers. Plant a garden.

4. Make a "joyful noise." Drown out the blues by listening to uplifting music. Sing along and you'll feel even better. Try Mozart. Researchers say the classical composer's music is mood-enhancing.

5. Keep a book of simple devotions (like *The Daily Word* or *Our Daily Bread*) or brief, uplifting stories (such as *A Cup of Chicken Soup for the Soul*) handy and read from it often, especially when you feel yourself slipping into depression. Turn to favorite passages in the Bible or read the Psalms if you're unfamiliar with Scripture. *Daily Light on the Daily Path,* a centuries-old collection of Scriptures in daily readings, is another good way of getting into the Bible.

6. Ask your friends of faith for prayer. Turn to your church pastor or prayer chain (consult the Yellow Pages or a friend if you don't attend a church). Ask your spouse to pray with you and for you if possible.

7. Write down some specific, affirming statements about your health and your life that you would like to see come to pass (i.e. "I am healthy in every way: mentally, physically and spiritually" or "I have many wonderful friends.") Say them aloud several times each day. Begin to act as if what you're saying is fact.

8. Seek counseling or treatment from a reputable psychologist, psychiatrist, homeopath, licensed clinical social worker or pastor. Enlist the help of a family member or friend in locating a physician or counselor.

9. Watch what you're eating. "Comfort" foods (like chocolate) are okay, in moderation. Increase protein and complex carbohydrate intake and decrease simple sugars and caffeine. Make sure to include enough monounsaturated fat or Omega-3 fatty acids in your diet. Your brain needs them. Consider vitamin and mineral supplements, especially B complex, C, D, potassium and magnesium. Don't try to self-medicate with herbs, and never take herbs in combination with prescription drugs. Get guidance from a reputable doctor or nutritionist. Avoid alcohol and recreational drugs like you would the plague! Warm milk or a relaxing bath beats a hot toddy at bedtime. Get help immediately if you can't sleep.

10. Remember that suicide is not the answer. It's the ultimate cop-out. God has a specific purpose for your life. You were created in His image. Just as day follows night, your pain will not last forever. Talk about your feelings instead of surrendering to thoughts of loneliness and despair.

Advice for a Family Member or Friend:

1. If you see obvious symptoms of stress burnout, excessive anxiety or depression, gently encourage the person to slow down or see a doctor. Talk to her and take the initiative to make a doctor's appointment, if necessary.

2. Encourage the depressed person to go out among people or into an environment that can stimulate him and break him out of inertia. Take him to lunch. Take her shopping. Listen to their concerns in a nonjudgmental way.

3. Accompany your loved one on a walk or join an exercise class together. Encourage participation in some kind of physical activity. Get creative if you have to. ("Could you help me move this piece of furniture ... stack this firewood ... plant these flowers?" etc.).

4. Tune the radio to an upbeat station or play an inspirational CD or tape in the background if a depressed person can't bring himself to do this. Let her hear you humming a happy tune now and then. Sounds silly? Try it.

5. Try sitting down with the person over a cup of tea or whatever you enjoy (preferably caffeine-free) and read out loud, as in the traditional family devotion time. Leave inspirational material lying around in prominent places or try books on tape.

6. Ask if you can pray for the depressed person. Take your loved one's hands or hold her in your arms and pray a loving, affirming prayer. If you're not comfortable or well-versed at prayer, remember a simple sentence or two will suffice. Just offer the love in your heart for this person to God. Hearing you do this can have a therapeutic effect on a depressed person.

7. Speak loving, affirming words to and about your depressed

loved one on every occasion you can. Help him to see himself as he can be. Remind him of the good times and assure him the sunshine will come back. Encourage her when you see improvement.

8. Many times a loved one needs a gentle push in the right direction in order to find help. Take her to the doctor and be there for support. Ask questions and get the information you need to help him help himself.

9. See to it that the right foods are on hand. Get actively involved with shopping and meal preparation, if necessary. Encourage the depressed person to prepare meals with you, to the extent that he or she can. Avoid too much fast food, a temptation if you're not a cook. If the depressed person is not eating and is losing weight, get him to a doctor. Antidepressant medication can restore the appetite. Curb your own alcohol consumption and take steps to ensure your loved one does the same. Remove alcohol from your house, if necessary.

10. Take any indications that the depressed person is considering suicide seriously. This is especially true in the case of senior citizens or adolescents. Remove from reach guns, razors, scissors, knives or drugs — anything with which he could harm himself, within reason. Encourage her to talk about suicidal feelings. Get *immediate* help from a crisis intervention center or the patient's doctor.

Notes

Introduction
1. Anne Frank: *The Diary of a Young Girl* (New York: Pocket Books, 1952); p. 177.

Chapter One
1. Title: Psalm 42:5 (King James Version)
2. Norman Vincent Peale; *How to Handle Tough Times* © 1990; Reprinted by permission of the Peale Center for Christian Living; p. 5.
3. Two-parent family data obtained from the Christian Coalition; 1995.
4. Pamela Kaney, "The Power of Music to Help and Heal," *Christian Counseling Today,* Fall 1998.
5. Prov 17:22
6. Excerpted from the book *A Quite Place in a Crazy World* by Joni Eareckson Tada; Multnomah Books; Questar Publishers; copyright 1993 by Joni Eareckson Tada; p 160.
7. Phil. 4:8
8. Prov. 23:7 (King James Version)
9. Prov. 18:21
10. Prov. 12:18.
11. Shad Helmstetter, Ph.D.; *The Self-talk Solution* (New York: Pocket Books, 1987); p. 17.
12. Bernie S. Siegel, M.D.; *Peace; Love and Healing* (New York: Harper & Row Publishers, 1989); p. 4.
13. Norman Cousins; *The Healing Heart* (New York: W.W. Norton & Company, 1983); p. 230.
14. Mark 8:36
15. 2 Cor. 12:9

Chapter Two
1. *Anne Frank: The Diary of a Young Girl*; p. 143
2. Henry David Thoreau; "Walking;" 1862; *Civil Disobedience and Other Essays* (Mineola, New York: Dover Publications, Inc., 1993); p. 49.

Chapter Three
1. *Depressive Illnesses: Treatments Bring New Hope;* 1993; U.S. Department of Health and Human Services (National Institute of Mental Health); p. 3.
2. Frank Bruno, Ph.D.; *Psychological Symptoms*; Copyright ©1993 by Frank Bruno, Ph.D. Reprinted by permission of John Wiley & Sons, Inc., New York.; p. 55.
3. Siegel; p. 158

4. Hara Estroff Marano; "Depression: Beyond Serotonin;" *Psychology Today*; March/April 1999; p. 72.
5. Bruno; *Op. Cit.*
6. Mark Gold, M.D.; *The Good News About Depression*; Rev. Ed. (New York: Bantam Books, 1995); p. 188.
7. Marano; *Op. Cit.*
8. Caryl Stern; "Why Depression is a Silent Killer;" *Parade* Magazine; Sept. 28, 1997; pp. 4- 5.
9. From the Surgeon General's announcement on suicide awareness and prevention as reported by the Associated Press on July 29, 1999.
10. *Ibid.*
11. C.G. Jung; "Dream Analysis in its Practical Application; "*Modern Man in Search of a Soul* (New York: Harcourt; Brace & World, Inc., 1933); p. 17.
12. David D. Burns, M.D.; *Feeling Good: The New Mood Therapy* (New York: William Morrow and Company Inc., 1980); p. 24.
13. Sharon Stocker; "Shelter Your Health From Emotional Stress;" *Prevention* Magazine; April 1994; p. 74.
14. *Ibid.*
15. Joannie M. Schrof and Stacey Schultz; "Melancholy Nation;" *U.S. News & World Report*; March 8, 1999; pp. 56-57.
16. Shad Helmstetter, Ph.D.; *Network of Champions* (Tucson, Arizona: Chapel & Croft Publishing, Inc.; 1995.); p. 77.
17. Gary Robertson; "Beating Depression;" *The News & Advance*, Lynchburg, Virginia; June 25, 1999, B-1.
18. Information obtained in an interview with Dr. James McCullough on July 6, 1999.
19. Jane Missett; "Analysis: Modern Psychiatry Shocking;" *North County Times*; Escondido, California; Feb. 9, 1997; E-5.
20. "10 Physical Reasons You May Be Depressed;" *Prevention* Magazine; June 1992; p. 70-76, p. 134.
21. *Our Daily Bread;* Radio Bible Class Ministries; 1996.
22. David Seamands; *Healing for Damaged Emotions*; (Colorado Springs, Colorado: Chariot Family Publishing, 1991); p. 123.
23. Earl Ubell; "Find Out if You Need Help;" *Parade ;*September 19, 1996; p. 16. Reprinted with permission from the author and *Parade* © 1996.
24. "Prevalence of Psychiatric Disorders Greater Than Previously Estimated;" *NIH Observer*; 4th Quarter 1994; p. 2, p. 11.
25. *Ibid.*
26. "Former Director of NIMH Says NIH-NIMH Reunion Signifies Importance of Brain and Behavior Research;" *NIH Observer;* 4th Quarter 1994; p. 15.

27. Schrof and Schultz; *Op. Cit.*
28. Jim Thornton; "Getting Inside Your Head;" *USA Weekend;* January 1-3, 1999; p. 6.
29. *The Complete Book of Vitamins*; Editors of *Prevention* Magazine (Emmaus, Pennsylvania: Rodale Press, 1984); p. 152, p. 456.
30. *Ibid.*
31. Michael T. Murray, N.D.; *Stress, Anxiety and Insomnia* (Prime Publishing, 1995)
32. Maxwell Maltz, M.D., F.I.C.S.; *Psycho-Cybernetics* (Paramus, New Jersey: Prentice-Hall Direct, 1960); pp. 78-79.
33. Marano, p. 33.
34. Phil. 4:6 (New American Standard Bible)
35. Prov. 3:5

Chapter Five

1. 1 Cor. 1:27b
2. 2 Cor. 12:9b
3. Barbara Johnson; *Fresh Elastic for Stretched-out Moms* (Grand Rapids, Michigan: Fleming H. Revell Publishing, 1985); p. 179
4. Eph. 6:4
5. Siegel; p. 176
6. James C. Dobson, Ph.D.; *Preparing for Adolescence* (Ventura, California: Regal Books, 1978, 1989).
7. Dr. Robert H. Schuller; *Self-Love* © 1969 by Jove Books; Reprinted by permission of Crystal Cathedral Ministries. All rights reserved; pp. 72-73.
8. *Ibid.*
9. From *Compassionate Capitalism* by Rich DeVos, copyright © 1993 by Compassionate Capitalism, Inc. Used by permission of Dutton, a division of Penguin Putnam Inc. (New York: Dutton); p. 42.
10. As reported on ABC "World News Tonight;" April 3, 1998.
11. Matt. 7:7
12. Peggy Noonan; "You'd Cry Too if it Happened to You;" *Forbes*, September 14, 1992; p. 58.
13. DeVos; p. 32
14. *Ibid.*
15. Seamands; p. 106.
16. Charles L. Whitfield; *Healing the Child Within* (Deerfield Beach, Florida: Health Communications, Inc., 1987); p. 101, p. 83.
17. DeVos; p. 34
18. Larry Crabb, Ph.D.; *Connecting* (Dallas: Word Publishing, 1998); pp. 191-192.
19. Carl Sandburg; "Aprons of Silence;" *Smoke and Steel* (New York: Harcourt Brace Jovanovich, Inc., 1936).

20. James Allen; *As a Man Thinketh* © 1904; Motivational Classics (1983); Life Management Services, Inc.; pp.118-119.
21. 2 Tim. 1:7
22. Peale; p. 62
23. Siegel; p. 198
24. *Ibid.*
25. Mark 14:34
26. *Our Daily Bread;* 1966

Chapter Six

1. Mark 12:30-31
2. Jung; "Psychotherapists or the Clergy;" *Modern Man in Search of a Soul;* p. 235.
3. Cal Thomas; *The Things That Matter Most* (New York: HarperCollins Publishers, Inc., Zondervon, 1994); p. 171.
4. Col. 2:8
5. Research data provided by Focus on the Family; 1998.
6. James C. Dobson, Ph.D.; *What Wives Wish Their Husbands Knew About Women;* © 1975 by Tyndale House Publishers, Inc., Wheaton, Illinois.; Eighth Printing; (Living Books, 1981); p. 25.
7. U.S. Department of Health and Human Services (Centers for Disease Control/National Center for Health Statistics); Tables for 1979-1995.
8. "Gonadal Steroids May Regulate Circadian Rhythms in Humans; Play Role in Developing Affective Disorders;" *NIH Observer*; 4th Quarter 1994; p. 5.
9. Bruno Bettelheim; *Surviving and Other Essays* (New York: Alfred A. Knopf, 1979); p. 106.
10. Heb. 2:7 (King James Version)
11. 1 John 4:4 (New American Standard Bible)
12. Phil. 4:13 (New American Standard Bible)
13. Herbert Benson, M.D.; *The Relaxation Response* (New York: Avon Books, 1975); p. 94.
14. Siegel; p. 119
15. Siegel; p. 124
16. Gary Smalley and John Trent, Ph.D.; *The Blessing* (New York: Pocket Books, 1986).
17. Excerpted from the book *The Prayer That Heals* by Francis MacNutt. Copyright 1981 by Ave Maria Press; Notre Dame, Indiana 46556; p. 106.
18. MacNutt; p. 107.
19. Luke 6:19
20. George Howe Colt; "The Magic of Touch," *Life;* August 1997; p. 60.
21. Colt; p. 61.
22. *Our Daily Bread*; 1996

23. Minister Ray McClendon; *Dr. Laura: A Mother in America* (Colorado Springs, Colorado: Chariot Victor Publishing, 1999), pp. 174-175.
24. Isaiah 57:15
25. Eccl: 3:2-4; 11a
26. Isaiah 57: 16a; 18a; 20-21
27. C. S. Lewis; *Mere Christianity* (New York: Macmillan Publishing Company, 1943); pp. 52-53.

Chapter Seven
1. Lourine M. Massie; "Fail Me Not;" 1962. Previously unpublished. Printed by permission of the author.

Chapter Eight
1. Prov. 6:32-33
2. James: 1:2-3
3. Romans 5:3-4
4. Lewis; *Op. Cit.*

Chapter Nine
1. Russell R. Thurman; "Moments of My Years;" 1981. Previously unpublished. Printed by permission of the author.

Chapter Ten
1. Jung; "Psychotherapists or the Clergy;" p. 226.
2. *Ibid.*
3. Jung; p. 228
4. Charles Allen; "When You Get the Blues;" Source unknown.
5. "The Natural;" Tri-Star Pictures, Inc.; 1984.
6. DeVos; p. 17.

Chapter Eleven
1. Norman Cousins; Source unknown. As reprinted in *Read and Grow Rich* by Burke Hedges © Burke Hedges and Steve Price (Tampa, Florida: INTI Publishing & Resource Books, Inc., 1999); p. 38.
2. Cousins; p. 129.
3. Edgar J. Scherick; "Write Yarns For Their Hungry Souls;" *ScreenWriter Quarterly*; Fall 1996; p. 50.
4. Mona Charen, "Cultural Indicators Not So Encouraging;" Syndicated column appearing in *The News & Advance,* Lynchburg, Virginia; Nov. 3, 1999; A-8.
5. Henry David Thoreau; *Walden and Other Writings;* Edited by Joseph Wood Krutch (New York: Bantam Books, 1962); p. 1.

6. Psalm 13:1-2
7. Frances Hodgson Burnett; *The Secret Garden* (1911); (Puffin Books, 1994); p. 146.
8. Kathy Cronkite; *On the Edge of Darkness* (New York: Bantam Doubleday Dell Publishing Group, Inc., 1994); p. 193.
9. Joel L. Swerdlow; "Vincent Van Gogh: Lullaby in Color;" *National Geographic*; October 1997; p. 106.
10. Ibid.
11. Ibid.
12. Swerdlow, p.112
13. Eugene O'Neill; *Long Day's Journey Into Night* © 1956; 33rd Printing; (New Haven: Yale University Press, 1975); p. 61.
14. O'Neill; p. 76.
15. O'Neill; p. 93.
16. Jane Austen; *Persuasion* (1818); (New York: Signet Classics/New American Library, 1964); p. 221.
17. James Boswell; *Life of Johnson*; Based on the third edition from 1799 (London/New York: Oxford University Press, 1953); pp. 115, 142, 216 and 315.
18. Boswell; p. 63.
19. Anthony Burgess; *The New York Times Book Review;* 1960.
20. Lewis; p. 124.
21. Harold S. Kushner; *Who Needs God* (New York: Simon & Schuster Inc., 1989); p. 40.
22. Romans 8:26
23. Institute of Creation Research; Santee, California (www.icr.org).
24. Sharon Begley with Marian Westley; "Science Finds God;" *Saturday Evening Post*; January-February 1999; p. 44.
25. Begley, p. 43.
26. Psalm 19:1
27. Psalm 19:11
28. 2 Peter: 1:4
29. Romans 15:4
30. Psalm 77:11
31. Deut. 8:2
32. Phil. 4:7 (New American Standard Bible)

Epilogue

1. Verses from Psalm 119: New American Standard Bible
2. Hugh Prather; *Notes on Love and Courage* (New York: Doubleday, 1977).
3. Phil. 1:6

Where To Get Information and Help

D/ART (Depression: Awareness, Recognition and Treatment)
ADEP (Anxiety Disorders Education Program),
National Institute of Mental Health (NIMH)
6001 Executive Blvd., Room 8184
Rockville, MD 20892-9663
(301) 443-4140
1-800-421-4211 or 1-888-826-9438 (free brochure)
www.nimh.nih.gov/dart or www.nimh.gov/anxiety

National Alliance for the Mentally Ill
Colonial Place Three
2107 Wilson Blvd.
Arlington, VA 22201
1-800-950-NAMI (6264)
www.nami.org

National Depressive and Manic Depressive Association
730 North Franklin Street, Suite 501
Chicago, IL 60610
1-800-DMDA (3632)
www.ndmda.org

National Foundation for Depressive Illness
P.O. Box 2257
New York, NY 10116
(212) 268-4260
1-800-248-4344 (information recording)
www.depression.org

National Mental Health Association
1021 Prince Street
Alexandria, VA 22314
1-800-969-NMHA (6642)
www.nmha.org

Unipolar Mood Disorders Institute (Research and Treatment)
Psychology Department, Virginia Commonwealth University
700 W. Grace Street
Suite 303
Richmond, VA 23220
(804) 828-5637

Focus on the Family
Colorado Springs, CO 80995
(719) 531-3400
Provides referrals through National Counseling Referral Network.
www.family.org

About the Author

Debbie Thurman makes her home in Central Virginia with her husband, Russ, and their two daughters, Jenni and Natalie. A native Virginian, she lived more than 17 years in San Diego County, California where her husband completed a 21-year, globe-spanning career in the U.S. Marine Corps. Debbie served as a Marine public affairs officer for eight years. She has worked in corporate communications and has been a freelance writer, magazine editor and a homeschool educator, among other endeavors. For speaking engagements or other information, the author can be reached through Cedar House Publishers at P.O. Box 399, Monroe, Virginia 24574-0399 or via e-mail at cedarhousepub@aol.com.